PRAISE FOR
ACHIEVING EQUILIBRIUM

"The guidance from this book, through the practice of Autogenic Therapy (AT), has immeasurably enhanced both my personal and professional life. AT should be a standard part, not only of every mental health professional's therapeutic toolkit, but recognised as a necessary resource for us as 'humans' to manage the inevitability of this often unsafe and uncertain world in which we live. *Achieving Equilibrium* is an eloquent, accessible, engaging manual that can be used across cultural, professional, and personal domains, to maintain our homeostasis."

Marianne Le Coyte Grinney, specialist family &
systemic psychotherapist and clinical lead

"I very much welcome *Achieving Equilibrium* as a comprehensive introduction to Autogenic Therapy. It provides a step-by-step guide to this powerful technique. This book is a useful tool, offering readers the opportunity to learn this deceptively simple technique, and allowing them to take control of their anxiety and stress, improving general wellbeing."

Shanagh Telford, homeopath

"*Achieving Equilibrium* is a very welcome book. Our world presents us with serious issues, all of which impact our wellbeing and cause us to experience stress in our bodies. The authors have given us a clear and comprehensive pathway using AT exercises to help us heal our bodies from the effects of this stress. As a psychotherapist and mindfulness teacher, I will be recommending this book to my clients as a tool to support their wellbeing and to manage and heal the symptoms of stress in their lives."

Maureen Treanor, psychotherapist, supervisor and mindfulness teacher

"As a doctor working with patients with sleep behaviour problems, I have found that patients who don't respond well to cognitive behaviour therapy can benefit from AT. I believe that readers of *Achieving Equilibrium* can benefit from learning AT, as it is a proven effective stress reduction process, and it is well known that many physical conditions improve once people have learned to profoundly relax."

Dr. Peter Gruenewald, MD, psychologist

"This volume will enable many to become aware of Autogenic Therapy in this year of the celebration of 100 years of AT's development and years to come. The authors are to be commended for providing both theoretical and practical insights into the many beneficial aspects of AT. I appreciate the comprehensive detailed Glossary, so good to have some details of the history and people who have been instrumental in the first 100 years of AT. It will be a pleasure to share copies with colleagues and friends."

Judith Wren, former British Autogenic Society chairperson

ACHIEVING EQUILIBRIUM

ACHIEVING EQUILIBRIUM

A Simple Way to Balance Body and Mind

Gaylin Tudhope and Ros Draper

AEON

First published in 2023 by
Aeon Books

British Library Cataloguing in Publication Data

A C.I.P. for this book is available from the British Library

ISBN-13: 978-1-80152-075-1

Illustrators: Helen Broadbridge and Ian Findlay
Typeset by Medlar Publishing Solutions Pvt Ltd, India

www.aeonbooks.co.uk

The greatest weapon against stress is our ability to choose one thought over another. Action seems to follow feeling, but really action and feeling go together, and by regulating the action, which is under the more direct control of the will, we can indirectly regulate the feeling which is not.

—William James
American Psychologist

The coordinated physiological processes which maintain most of the steady states in the organism are so complex and so peculiar to living beings—involving, as they may, the brain and nerves, the heart, lungs, kidneys and spleen, all working cooperatively—that I have suggested a special designation for these states homeostasis. The word does not imply something set and immobile, a stagnation. It means a condition— a condition which may vary but which is relatively constant. Homeostasis describes the adaptive mechanisms that preserve functional stability in the face of environmental change. Great emotional stress could trigger uncontrolled hormonal secretion, particularly from the pituitary, thyroid and adrenal glands, which would play havoc with our internal adjustments and lead to disease.

—Walter Cannon
American Physiologist

*Once the body achieves a state of neuromuscular homeostasis
the mind will follow suit.*

—Edmund Jacobson
American Physician

*Stress like relativity is a scientific concept, which has suffered from
the mixed blessing of being too well known and too little understood.
Man should not try to avoid stress any more than he would shun food,
love or exercise. It is not stress that kills us, it's our reaction to it.
Adopting the right attitude can convert a negative stress into a positive one.*

—Hans Selye
Hungarian-Canadian Endocrinologist

*Self regulation depends on having a friendly relationship with your body.
Without it you have to rely on external regulation—from medication,
drugs like alcohol, constant reassurance, or compulsive compliance with
the wishes of others. Neuroscience research shows that the only way we
can change the way we feel is by becoming aware of our inner experience
and learning to befriend what is going on inside ourselves.*

—Bessel van der Kolk
Dutch-American Psychiatrist

*The research literature has identified three factors that universally lead to
stress: uncertainty, the lack of information and the loss of control. Well
self-regulated people are the most capable of interacting fruitfully with
others in a community and of nurturing children who will also grow
into self-regulated adults. Anything that interferes with that natural
agenda threatens the organism's chances for long-term survival.*

—Gabor Mate
Hungarian-Canadian Physician

Because of what's called experience-dependent neuroplasticity whatever you hold in attention has a special power to change your brain. Controlling your attention—becoming more able to place it where you want it and keep it there ... is the foundation of changing your brain, and thus your life, for the better. As the great psychologist William James wrote over a century ago 'The education of attention would be the education par excellence'.

—*Rick Hanson*
American Neuropsychologist

CONTENTS

PART 2
BACKGROUND INFORMATION

PART 3
THE HISTORY OF AUTOGENICS

PART 4
CASE STUDIES

Medical matters
When is AT treatment recommended by the medical
    profession
Medical questionnaire uses
Case studies pain management, high blood pressure,
    dermatological problems, anxiety

ABOUT THE AUTHORS

The authors are two psychotherapists with many years of experience working with individuals, couples, families, and organisations. Naturally, we each have a different story about our relationship with and experience of autogenic training (AT).

Gaylin: I completed my AT training in 1998 and as an AT trainer and practitioner I have trained numerous people around the world. I believe strongly that daily use of AT has enormous health benefits and I collaborate with many GPs whose patients with stress-related symptoms such as anxiety, high blood pressure, and sleep issues are helped through learning AT practice with me. The healing power of AT always astounds me each time I teach it and use it.

Ros: I began learning AT in 2019 and was so impressed with the healing potential of AT that in 2020 I undertook the BAS (British Autogenic Society) AT training. I have found AT practice to have enormous health benefits personally and now recommend AT to many of my clients. My wish is for more people to know about this wonderful self-care skillset which fits completely with my belief as a psychotherapist that there is an innate drive towards healing and health in every human being.

We (Gaylin and Ros), along with other AT practitioners, feel that AT urgently needs to be more accessible to a wider public and not only to those who can pay for training with a qualified AT practitioner. So this book offers people the possibility of teaching themselves the six AT standard exercises. We are convinced AT has substantial health benefits to cope with and navigate the demands of today's world.

FOREWORD

Dr Geoffrey Leader MB ChB FRCA Dip ION
Lucille Leader Dip ION CNHC Reg

We congratulate the authors of this book, Gaylin Tudhope and Ros Draper, on their presentation of the art and science of autogenic training (AT). It is academically based, yet in a practical, comprehensive format, easy to understand and apply to life situations. Their mission to enable calm and relaxed focus is accomplished.

AT plays a vital role, not only in integrated medical, para-medical, and psychological management, but also in everyday life situations. Whatever the need for spontaneous decision-making, whether it be general, business, or academic, or in health issues, these challenges can be optimally supported by the application of AT techniques acquired by training.

These specialised techniques, described by the authors in their easy-to-follow text, allow for the feeling of being 'centred', calm, and relaxed, and can then become part of spontaneous responses and decision-making by the individual. AT is eminently suitable for adults. It is also invaluable for children to acquire its techniques in order to support them during the stress of life's educational challenges, as well as with interpersonal relationships during youth and adulthood.

We have introduced the acquisition of AT techniques and their application to children who have thereafter reported better control of stress at exam times and when confronted with personal and sleep issues. We have had the pleasure of including autogenic training in our integrated medical management clinics for patients with chronic illnesses and also for their carers. This has been presented to our patients by Gaylin Tudhope, psychologist and co-author of this book.

Feedback from patients has been exceptional and they are appreciative of the tools gained to enable better management of their stress, anxiety, medical symptoms, and sleep problems—the latter facilitating body regenerative processes. However, as the authors of this book have highlighted, it is important for people with significant chronic illnesses to consult their integrated medical team before commencing a course of AT training.

We have great pleasure in recommending this book to all individuals who wish to acquire calmness and relaxation. The helpful techniques presented are logical and easy to understand.

PREFACE

The idea for this book emerged in 2020 during the early stages of the COVID-19 pandemic that has affected people in all corners of the globe as we realised how important it is for as many people as possible to have easy access both to an understanding of the health value of Autogenics and instructions for learning and practising Autogenics. Specifically, we wanted to provide people with a way to teach themselves the six AT standard exercises, which are the core of Autogenics, without having to rely on professional help. Indeed, it was the vision of Johannes Schulz, the creator of Autogenics, that people be able to use this self-care skillset without the need to depend on a professional they had to pay. With this book, we want people to be able to teach themselves the basics of Autogenics.

Both of us authors are experienced psychotherapists who, through practising Autogenics ourselves, share a conviction that understanding and learning about Autogenics can help anyone interested in optimising their capacity for self-regulation of their body mind system. In this book we hope we explain how understanding this innate capacity of our body mind system means we can at will activate our parasympathetic nervous system—our rest, repair, restore, and relax mechanism. It is knowing how to self-regulate that enables us to maintain physical and emotional balance in the inner and outer worlds of our body mind system, which is an essential ingredient of self-care. So it follows that we wanted to find a way to share the information necessary for people to teach themselves the six AT standard exercises, which we know can enhance our wellbeing and strengthen our resilience.

We could see from our own work with our clients since the beginning of the COVID-19 pandemic that many people have become more and more aware of the everyday stressors to their autonomic nervous system (ANS) created by the pandemic and are therefore recognising the importance of having a repertoire of skills for taking care of their wellbeing. We also already knew from our own experience of regular daily practice of the six standard exercises that Autogenics has a very important part to play in self-care, the promotion of wellbeing, the strengthening of our immune system, and we believe in disease prevention. We wanted therefore to make the six AT standard exercises available to anyone who would read this book so as to increase their sense of agency as they focus on their self-care, maintenance, and promotion of their own wellbeing and resilience during these most challenging 21st century times.

In this book, we want to convey our conviction that knowing how to use the six AT standard exercises can provide us all with direct access, when professional help maybe unavailable or unaffordable, to a means of restoring balance to our body mind system. When our nervous system (ANS) is out of balance, there is a greater potential for illness as our immune system can become compromised by chronic stress. By restoring the balance (homeostasis) needed between our sympathetic (SNS) and parasympathetic (PSNS) nervous systems, we create conditions for our body mind system to self-regulate, thereby minimising the impact of adverse experiences and the unavoidable imbalances stressors create in our autonomic nervous system (ANS).

We say unavoidable imbalances because life always has its up and downs with bumps in the road. Autogenics is a skill-set that helps us navigate these bumps and restore the balance which is vital for the robust body mind system we need if we are to be able to bounce back from adverse experiences. It is this balance (homeostasis) that provides us with the highway to wellbeing and it is our body mind system's innate capacity to self-regulate, which is the core idea that we want our book to get across to readers.

We are all born with this capacity to self-regulate and just need to understand how we can with intention tap into this innate capacity as we journey through life, navigating more or less stress due to the inevitable internal and external stressors we all regularly experience.

Predictably, partly because of our own ongoing work commitments and the honing of our thinking about how best to present these ideas, we encountered delays as we worked on the book and we now find ourselves writing this preface in April 2022.

Spring 2022, when we are writing this preface, turns out to be the year of the Russian invasion and war with Ukraine, which is an additional stressor to our nervous systems (ANS) already on high alert, whether we are conscious of this or not, from the effects of two years of living with the pandemic. Among the people we meet, we see a continuum of the different ways we can react to the 'bad news' either with denial, e.g. wars are a long way away and won't affect us … or with paralysing fear, e.g. we may be about to be reduced to dust by an atomic bomb, and anywhere in between those two extremes. Given everyone's nervous system (ANS) is being impacted in some way by anxieties, regarding climate change, wars, global disease infections, and economic hardships, where would you place yourself on the continuum—paralysed by fear or in denial or somewhere in between?

We believe it is important for our ongoing self-care and wellbeing to understand where on the continuum our own reactions at any given time to tragic and frightening news place us. However, it is as important that regardless of our responses to the impact of say the present war in Ukraine, we all recognise our need to know how to protect our body mind systems and to self-regulate. In the face of any adverse experiences that activate our sympathetic nervous system—our fight, flight, freeze response, our ability to self-regulate—both our physical and mental wellbeing is affected. Self-regulation and resilience are close cousins that help us cope with stress and adapt to change as well as support our wellbeing and self-esteem.

Learning the six AT standard exercises as described in this book will help anyone, whether impacted by war or less dramatic bumps in the road we call life, learn and know how to self-regulate. AT is therefore a reliable resource for the promotion of health and wellbeing available to us all if we set aside the time to learn the six AT standard exercises, so we have a skillset that we can use anywhere and at any time.

Our fervent wish is for people reading this book to feel empowered not just in an emergency situation when Autogenics is definitely helpful but to know they are able to self-regulate before, during, and after any difficult situations they may encounter. It is our hope that once people have experienced and understood the homeostatic balancing effect of self-regulation they will be determined to hold onto the knowledge of how to activate this innate capacity available to all human beings as part of their self-care repertoire.

In order to reach the maximum number of readers in an era of audio books and apps, we have arranged the sections of the book so that if you just want to learn the six AT standard exercises there is a discreet section with all the information you need plus links to video recordings you may want to use as prompts as you are learning. If, on the other hand, you are interested in the ideas behind Autogenics, some of the history and development worldwide of Autogenics, there are sections in the book with this information. We have also included a section where we offer answers to questions we and others have asked as we have worked with Autogenics, as well as a section with some case studies. Each section is discreet and stand-alone.

We acknowledge there are other books about Autogenics as well as online resources available many of which go beyond what we are calling the basics. However, we hope rather boldly perhaps that this book, aiming as it does to provide a way for readers to teach themselves the basic ideas and practices of the six AT standard exercises without needing input from a professional, can make a significant contribution to the self-care literature. If readers' appetites are whetted to learn more, so much the better.

Gaylin Tudhope and Ros Draper
England, 2022

INTRODUCTION

This book introduces readers to autogenic training (AT), which like its name, auto = self and genic = generating—self generating, means that it allows for self regulating of the mind and body. AT is a unique self-help tool created in the 1920s by Johannes Schulz, a German physician. AT is for those of us concerned about learning a skillset that can help us optimise and support our resilience as well as restore our health and wellbeing anytime we develop symptoms in response to stressors in our lives. For health maintenance, we each need to recognise what causes negative stress to our body mind system and also to learn how to insulate ourselves from the effects of these stressors. It is our belief that understanding and being able to use AT, via the six AT standard exercises we are offering in this book, provides us with this much-needed insulation.

Offering this book at this time is part of our response to the many challenges we are all facing in the changed world of the 2020s and because we know AT can contribute to helping us successfully navigate unfamiliar territory without undue damage or suffering to our body mind systems. Early 21st-century challenges, whether from the adaptations required by the pandemic, the consequences of wars, daily working in front of a screen, or commutes to and from an office, mean our body mind systems are exposed to many different stressors.

Practising AT regularly can mitigate some of the bodily stress from sitting at a computer for prolonged periods of time. Practising AT regularly can also mitigate the effects, which of course vary from individual to individual, of constant exposure to news and information good and bad via electronic platforms.

As the 20th century progressed, health professionals increasingly emphasised the need to learn self-care, calming, and self-soothing skillsets to counteract the effects of everyday stressors; put another way, how to learn to access our body mind system's inbuilt relaxation response. So today, healthcare practitioners of both conventional allopathic Western medicine as well as functional, alternative, or complementary medicine practitioners routinely assess a patient's understanding of, relationship with, and motivation for acquiring self-care skills.

AT can sit comfortably alongside popular, effective, well-documented, and researched self-care skillsets, like meditation, tracking heart rate variability, yoga, massage, BioFeedback, swimming, breathwork, hiking, walking, and other pursuits, all of which can support our wellbeing. What we believe distinguishes AT from other self-care skillsets is that its goal is to directly activate the body mind system's own inbuilt capacity for self-regulation. It is self-regulation that promotes or restores the balance (homeostasis) our body mind system needs in order for relaxation, rest, and repair to happen or for our parasympathetic nervous system to be activated so our resilience can be supported and maintained. It is this innate capacity for self-regulation that triggers the relaxation response in our body mind system. Relaxation is therefore a by-product of a body mind system in balance so not the primary goal of practising the six AT standard exercises.

AT then refers to the way in which our mind can influence our body and our body influence our mind to come to a state of balance (homeostasis) in which the inbuilt self-regulating capacity of our autonomic nervous system (ANS) can do its job. This balance can occur only when our sympathetic nervous system (SNS)—our fight, flight, freeze protective mechanism and our parasympathetic nervous system (PSNS)—our rest, restore, digest, and repair mechanisms are working in tandem to enable balance (homeostasis) for the wellbeing of our body mind system. Thus AT provides a way to enhance the positive and mitigate the negative effects of the inevitable stressors we encounter in life. Of course, each of us has a different threshold for tolerating levels of stress. So only when stress starts affecting our physical and mental wellbeing do we know our sympathetic nervous systems (SNS) has taken over. It is then that we need a skillset like AT so we are able to activate our parasympathetic nervous system (PSNS) in order to bring our body mind system back into balance.

AT is a series of easy to learn mental exercises for self-use designed to restore this balance (homeostasis) to our autonomic nervous system (ANS). Regular daily use of the six AT standard exercises enables us to turn off the sympathetic nervous system's (SNS) fight, flight, or freeze mechanism, which is designed and needed to deal with any real or perceived danger or threat we encounter, and turn on the parasympathetic nervous system (PSNS), which is designed and needed for repair, restoration, and relaxation of our body mind system. It is when these two systems, together with the enteric nervous system (ENS), are in a state of balance (homeostasis) that the inbuilt capacity of our ANS to regulate our body mind system can function efficiently—do the job it (ANS) was designed to do for us.

In the 21st century, it is now widely recognised by health professionals that it is our capacity for self-regulation of our autonomic nervous system (ANS) that is an important factor in the prevention and/or mitigation of the severity of many physiological and psychological problems and resilience building. What is less well known is that we can learn by regular use of the six AT standard exercises to access our body mind system's inbuilt capacity for this self-regulation. So AT, whilst not necessarily a cure for any condition and not aiming to replace standard medical treatments, can nevertheless help people better manage symptoms. This means people who practise AT and who are sufferers of anxiety-based disorders, post-traumatic stress disorder (PTSD), eating disorders, and even some learning disorders such as ADHD, to mention a few, can have an improved quality of life.

We aim with this book to enable readers to have easy access to the information they need to learn how to be able to switch at will from a body mind state dominated by the activity of the sympathetic nervous system (SNS) to a state in which the parasympathetic system (PSNS) is doing its job of rest, relaxation, and repair. Knowing how to restore body mind balance (homeostasis) prevents us from getting stuck in the overactive state of the sympathetic nervous system (SNS). It is the prolonged or chronic overactive body mind system state of the sympathetic nervous system (SNS) that can lead to anxiety, depression, insomnia, exhaustion, and other stress-related conditions, which in turn can effect vital body organs. Navigating this increasingly challenging and complex world of ours requires us to have a repertoire of skills to help us cope with stressors and adapt to change if we are to protect our mental and emotional wellbeing and remain resilient.

When practised daily, the six AT standard exercises provide a self-help skillset that promotes resilience, as practising AT calms the sympathetic nervous system (SNS), which is our body mind system's default neural network. This default network is constantly on the alert for perceived or actual threat but needs the parasympathetic nervous system (PSNS) to be on line too if we are to effectively manage stress, adapt to change, and maintain our resilience and wellbeing. When our sympathetic and parasympathetic mechanisms are working together and balanced, there is a reduction in symptoms of stress: anxiety, insomnia, dangerously high blood pressure, nausea, etc. as these and other symptoms are generally a consequence of imbalances in our body mind system when our self-regulating capacity is under functioning or compromised.

As well as introducing the reader to the six AT standard exercises, which are the foundation of AT as developed by the originator Johannes Schulz, we describe the background and development internationally of AT; how AT works to balance our body mind system; how to teach yourself the six AT standard exercises; how to access more AT resources in person or on line.

Recognising we all have different learning and reading styles, we have structured the book so there are four main sections and it is possible to dip in and out of the book depending on your interests. The four main stand-alone sections together give an overview of the theory and practice of AT.

However, anyone just wanting to learn the six AT standard exercises will find all they need in Part 1, where we introduce, describe, and give instructions for learning the six AT standard exercises for you to learn, practise, and use daily.

We include in Part 1 detailed information on how we need to prepare ourselves for AT practice: a brief body scan, using our dominant arm as a helpful cue for our body mind system to access the relaxation response, which means going into a Theta brainwave state, how to keep ourselves in a state of passive concentration/awareness, the various body postures recommended for use when practising the six AT standard exercises, plus the cancel, which is the final step in each AT practice session.

For anyone who learns best with audio-visual cues, there are accompanying videos (accessed via a token when you purchase the book) which Gaylin has made of the complete sequence of the six AT standard exercises in a format to be accessed week by week over the eight-week period recognised as an optimal way to learn AT. Once learnt, however, AT is best practised when we silently and interiorly repeat the exercise formulae to ourselves without the use of prompts from someone else. AT is a self-care skillset!

A video guide to Autogenics
https://vimeo.com/showcase/9750652

Part 2 is structured in the form of answers to questions each of us have asked at different times as we learnt to work with AT. When not to use AT (contraindications) is one of the questions we address in Part 2 as well as throughout the book, as it is vital that people with certain medical conditions only learn AT in consultation with a qualified AT practitioner.

In Part 3, we describe the history and international development of AT. This section includes descriptions of people, places, and ways in which professionals from different disciplines and in many different countries on all five continents have and are continuing to demonstrate the importance of AT as a self-help skillset.

In Part 4, we review common diseases encountered by medical practitioners whose patients have benefitted from the use of AT either as a stand-alone treatment intervention or alongside other treatments. We also include four case studies of familiar everyday disease situations where AT has been helpful in symptom relief with patients reporting becoming calmer, more focussed and less stressed, as well as a reduction in symptoms.

There are of course other resources already available for learning AT, and we list some of them in the section at the end of the book, along with some references for anyone wishing to explore and read more about AT.

We have put the 'Glossary of terms' relevant to AT and used throughout this book at the beginning of the text so you can easily reference any unfamiliar terms as you read.

Our hope is that you will want to learn AT which we believe in a few weeks can benefit your whole body mind system. More than that, if practising the six AT standard exercises whets you're appetite for more that you will want to explore in consultation with a qualified AT practitioner other applications of AT that can promote your wellbeing and contribute to your health maintenance.

GLOSSARY OF TERMS

Afferent refers to nerve fibres that carry signals from the periphery of our body towards the central nervous system (CNS) to the spinal cord, brain stem and our sensory processing systems, e.g. what we see, hear, smell, taste, touch, etc.

Autogenic discharge refers to involuntary reactions or side effects generated whilst doing the six AT standard exercises in response to your body mind system's need to offload sources of inner tension, such as:

- Effects of illness, injury, or accident
- Repressed emotions
- Repressed reactions
- Effects of intoxicating substances such as drug taking

Autogenic formulae is used interchangeably with the six AT standard exercises, and the word formulae is a direct translation from Johannes Schulz's (originator of AT) German texts on AT.

Autogenic process refers to the way AT enables the body mind system to access a Theta brainwave state that in turn allows for the body mind system to rebalance often leading to profound changes in physical and mental states and enhanced wellbeing.

Autogenic state refers to the particular state of consciousness induced by the practise of the six AT standard exercises as our body mind system becomes deeply relaxed. The practise of AT allows for us to reach this Theta space or access the relaxation response, which enables the body and brain to rebalance, activating our inbuilt capacity for homeostasis.

Autogenic training (AT) consists of a series of six mental exercises (in the text referred to as six AT standard exercises) which elicit the bodily sensations of warmth and heaviness, which in turn cue the body mind system into the psycho-physiological changes of the relaxation response.

Autonomic nervous system (ANS) regulates the internal environment of our bodies controlling our internal organs and glands, and is considered to be outside the realm of voluntary control. The ANS can be divided into the PSNS = parasympathetic nervous system, SNS = sympathetic nervous system, and ENS = enteric nervous system.

Autogenic training diary is something you will be asked to keep if you learn AT with a qualified practitioner, in order to discuss symptoms, discharges, and changes you may experience during your AT practice. A training diary is something you can keep for yourself to note any physical and emotional changes and to reflect on what is happening to you as you learn and practise AT.

Body mind system refers to the intricate and inseparable relationship between the body and the mind and resists the Western traditions of mind–body Cartesian split. For example, the endocrine and immune systems with all the organs of our body, together with all the emotional responses we have, share a common chemical language and are constantly communicating with one another.

Body scan in AT involves mentally paying attention to parts of the body and bodily sensations moving from feet to head or from head to feet in a sequence lasting approximately 60 seconds. With this mental scanning, we bring our awareness to every single part of our bodies, noticing any aches, pains, tensions, or general discomfort in preparation for our AT practice.

Body postures there are three standard postures recommended for autogenic training: horizontal posture (HP), simple sitting posture (SS), and reclining armchair posture (AP). These are recommended postures as each one can reduce afferent and efferent impulses, thus promoting maximum muscle relaxation during AT training.

Brainwave states, neural oscillations or brainwaves observed by researchers first in 1924, are rhythmic or repetitive patterns of neural activity in the central nervous system. Oscillatory activity in the brain is widely observed at different levels of organisation and is thought to play a key role in processing neural information.

Central nervous system (CNS) controls most functions of the body and mind system. The CNS consists of bundles of nerves in the brain and spinal cord that carry messages to and from the peripheral nervous system (PNS). The brain has a central role in the control of most bodily functions, whilst some reflex movements can occur via spinal cord pathways without the participation of brain structures.

Collective trauma refers to the psychological reactions to traumatic events shared by a group of people of any size, up to and including an entire society. People don't need to have experienced an event first hand, e.g. twin towers, the attack on Pearl Harbour, Holocaust, etc., to experience trauma, which can frequently lead to the development of intergenerational mental health problems.

Contraindications are any physical, emotional or mental conditions, characteristics, or symptoms that suggest a given treatment intervention is risky, inadvisable, or that there may be a poor outcome for the patient.

Distress is an unpleasant emotion, feeling, thought, condition, or behaviour which can affect the way we think, feel, or act and can create great anxiety, trouble, worry, and strain, sometimes accompanied by mental anguish and suffering.

Dominant arm the right or left side that we prefer for most tasks is known as the dominant arm or hand. We tend to say I am right or left handed as the dominant arm is more skilled in general, due to a combination of genetic predisposition and accumulated practice. In AT practice saying my right/left arm is heavy is the cue for the body mind system to switch into the Theta brainwave state.

Efferent refers to nerve fibres that carry impulses away from the brain or spinal cord to muscles, glands, other organs or cells, e.g. an artery is an efferent vessel that carries blood away from the heart.

Enteric nervous system (ENS) is known as the 'second brain' or the brain in the gut as it controls gastrointestinal behaviour independently of the central nervous system (CNS) and can also be influenced by the ANS.

Heart rate variability is a measure of the variation in time between each heartbeat and is controlled by the autonomic nervous system (ANS). High heart rate variability means the body is responsive to both parasympathetic (PANS) and sympathetic (SNS) mechanisms so the nervous system is balanced. A balanced nervous system (ANS) means the body mind system is capable of adapting with ease to its environment and performing at its best.

Homeostasis is a state of balance/equilibrium in which biological functions such as blood pressure and body temperature are maintained at an optimal level by the continuous adjustment of cells, tissues, and organisms inside the body to external and internal stimuli so that the body functions healthily. The complementary functions of the PSNS and SNS working in tandem maintain the body's homeostasis.

Hyperarousal is a primary symptom of PTSD and occurs when a person's body suddenly kicks into high alert as a result of thinking about previous trauma even though real danger may not be present.

Hypoarousal, also known as the 'freeze' response, is when a person feels shut down, numb, separate from his/her thoughts and feelings, disconnected from what is happening in the present. Dissociation, a characteristic of hypo arousal, usually happens when disconnecting from a traumatic event or memory of a traumatic event seems to be the only way to cope with helplessness, fear or pain.

Immune system is a complex network of cells, tissues, organs, and the substances they produce that helps the body fight invaders such as viruses, bacteria, foreign bodies, and other diseases.

Individual trauma occurs when an event, one-off, repeated, or chronic, that is emotionally painful or distressing is experienced as abnormally intense or stressful with effects on physical and mental health which are adverse and long-lasting.

Motor pathways are the part of the central nervous system (CNS) which allows for the movement of signals from the brain to the body and vice versa. They enable effective communication from brain to body and from body to brain.

Parasympathetic nervous system (PSNS) is the mechanism for activating bodily functions for repair, relaxation, rest, and digest that, in the absence of danger, slows the stress responses of the sympathetic nervous system (SNS) by automatically releasing hormones that relax the mind and body whilst inhibiting, or slowing, many of the high energy functions of the body (the PSNS dilates pupils, inhibits salivation, increases heart rate, dilates bronchi, inhibits digestion, inhibits contraction of the bladder).

Passive concentration is often the most challenging part of the autogenic training process as it requires you to 'observe' yourself focussing on each arm or leg or body part *without* trying to make anything happen.

Peripheral nervous system (PNS) is comprised of all parts of the nervous system nerves and groups of nerve cells (neurons) called ganglia lying outside of the brain and spinal cord.

Polyvagal theory developed by Dr Stephen Porges maintains the autonomic nervous system (ANS) produces three possible elementary states in response to internal and external stimuli experienced by the body mind system: *rest and digest* = social and safe; *fight-or-flight* = mobilisation; or *freeze, faint, or shutdown* = immobilisation. By focussing on what is happening in the body and the autonomic nervous system, we can see and monitor how our sense of safety or danger or threat impacts our behaviour.

Psycho-physiological shift refers to the continuous two-way flow of information from soma (body) to psyche (mind) and from psyche (mind) to soma (body)—as the six AT standard exercises bring about changes in our physiology, changes in our psyche also occur.

Relaxation response, a term first used by Herbert Benson in 1975, is the opposite of your body mind system's stress response (SNS) and describes a physical state of deep rest that can occur when the body mind system is no longer in perceived danger.

REM sleep is a kind of sleep that usually occurs within the first 90 minutes of falling asleep and then at intervals during the night and is characterised by rapid eye movements (REM), more dreaming, more bodily movement, faster pulse, and irregular breathing than recorded in other dream states. During REM sleep, our brain is almost as active as when we are awake.

Resilience is the ability to maintain or regain mental health despite experiencing adversity or to withstand adversity to recover and bounce back from difficult life events. Thus some people can be knocked down by life but come back stronger than ever. (resilience is different from mental toughness ... all mentally tough individuals are resilient, but not all resilient individuals are mentally tough).

Sensory pathways are responsible for the perception of sensations in our body and mind. They include those routes which take information to the conscious cortex of the brain. This is how we notice and feel sensations.

Self-regulation in autogenic practice refers to the body mind system's inbuilt capacity to manage disruptive impulses, emotions, and imbalances in our body chemistry, such as extreme or high adrenalin surges. Self-regulation restores homeostasis to the body mind system.

Somatic nervous system is that part of the peripheral nervous system that controls voluntary body movement through skeletal muscles. Afferent and efferent nerves are found in our somatic nervous system.

Standard AT exercises are the six exercises we learn for our auto-genic practice and are the basis of autogenic training. They are based on an exercise format created by Johannes Schultz and Wolfgang Luthe. The six AT standard exercises focus on:

- Heaviness—muscular relaxation
- Warmth cardiac regulation
- Respiration
- Warmth in the abdominal region
- Coolness in the cranial region

Stress is a term used by the endocrinologist Hans Selye in the 1920s to refer to human bodily responses designed to protect us from real or perceived danger. When working as intended, stress can help us stay energetic and alert. In an emergency, when fight, flight, or freeze is required, our stress responses can save us from danger. However, after a certain point, stress stops being helpful and can cause damage to our productivity, our immune system, our moods and emotions, and our general quality of life.

Sympathetic nervous system (SNS) is a survival mechanism that automatically prepares the body for the fight, flight, freeze, faint, or submit response when we encounter danger or there is a perceived threat to us. In the 21st century, we often have the same stress responses to non-life-threatening stressors of everyday life that can cause high levels of anxiety (the SNS constricts pupils, stimulates salivation, slows heart rate, constricts bronchi, stimulates digestion, causes the bladder to contract).

The cancel refers to the final stage of each AT exercise sequence. Named 'the cancel' because it is the way we come out of the relaxed autogenic state, as we need to be fully alert to resume our daily activities.

Theta brainwave state is the barely conscious state just before sleeping and just after waking … the border between the conscious and the unconscious. Whilst in the Theta state, the body mind system is capable of deep and profound learning, healing and growth.

Trapezius muscle is a muscle that starts at the base of the neck, goes across the shoulders, and extends to the middle of the back. The trapezius helps the movement of the head, neck, arms, shoulders, and torso, as well as stabilising the spine and helping with posture

Vagal tone results from the activity of the vagus nerve and is a mostly unconscious internal biological process. Increasing vagal tone activates the parasympathetic nervous system so having a higher vagal tone means the body can relax faster after experiencing stress. A high vagal tone is also associated with lower blood pressure, improved blood-sugar regulation, improved digestion, better mood, reduced anxiety, and reduced risk of stroke and cardiovascular disease. Healthy vagal tone is synonymous with emotional regulation.

Vagus nerve (vagus in Latin meaning wandering) is one of the longest nerves of the autonomic nervous system (ANS), connecting the brainstem to the body and helping to regulate heart rate, blood pressure, sweating, digestion, and even speaking.

Wellbeing is a broad concept used in respect to the physical and mental health of a person who feels good in and about her or himself, is functioning well with high level of life satisfaction, with a sense of meaning or purpose and has the ability to manage stress.

PART 1

THE SIX AT STANDARD EXERCISES

The six AT standard exercises are best learnt over an eight-week period, and in this book we offer you a format for each exercise with the heading 'Week 1—First standard exercise' and so on through the eight weeks.

We make suggestions for how you can manage your AT practice in Week 1, Week 2, and so on through the eight weeks. You can of course go more slowly to suit your own pace. However, we do not advise contracting your learning of the exercises to less than eight weeks.

Experience shows that in order for you to gain maximum benefit and reliably develop new neural pathways your body mind system needs the eight-week time span to learn and become familiar with the exercises. In other words, to develop a new habit.

With the instructions for each exercise, we also offer an explanation and the rationale for each of the exercises describing how they connect to bodily functions relevant to accessing your innate capacity for self-regulation, maintaining balance (homeostasis) in your body mind system, and improving vagal tone.

Along with the instructions for each of the six AT standard exercises, we list physical conditions or ailments which may be contraindications for each exercise. It is necessary for anyone with any of the conditions or ailments we list to always learn AT with a qualified AT practitioner who can monitor your progress and responses to the exercises week by week.

We know from experience that practising AT can in a few weeks benefit your whole body mind system. So whether you learn AT by teaching yourself the six standard exercises from this book or learn with a qualified AT practitioner we hope what you have read so far has whetted your appetite to continue reading!

Essential preparation for autogenic training

Autogenic environment

When beginning to learn AT you need a quiet atmosphere, as this will help the development of your capacity for passive concentration and awareness. It is helpful to remove your shoes, wear loose clothing, or loosen your clothing, so you feel comfortable. It is also important if you wear glasses to remove them during your AT practice.

AT practice is always best done when it is as quiet as possible. Later, when AT has become an established part of your daily routine, you may find it is possible to practise in most everyday situations, e.g. in a supermarket queue, at your office, on a bus or train, etc., without being distracted. Over time you will increasingly become able to shut out all external noise and be able to do your AT practice even in places where there are people and noise.

WARNING: YOU MUST NEVER ATTEMPT TO PRACTISE AT WHILST DRIVING A CAR OR OTHER VEHICLE.

Your autogenic training diary

Keeping a daily record of your AT practice is an important part of your autogenic training. Whilst optional, a diary does provide you with a record of your progress and allows you to reflect on your experiences as you learn and practise the six AT standard exercises. Your diary also allows you to chart your progress by developing clarity of observation with detachment. Your diary may also be used to record dreams or any unusual experiences that may occur at times when you are not doing AT.

Whether or not you manage three sessions daily, it is a good habit to make three entries daily in your diary. Then if you did not do all three AT practise sessions, you can write yourself an explanation of why you missed a practise session! This can be a fascinating exercise in its own right. Very quickly, you begin to see how effortlessly we can all fall into sabotaging our efforts to build the three daily AT exercise sessions into our daily routine.

The body scan

Always begin your AT practice by doing a quick (approximately 60 seconds) body scan starting either from the top of your head going downwards to your toes or from your toes travelling upwards to the top of your head. You can use any wording you wish and the body scan wording here is the same wording used on the video recordings, which you may want to access:

A video guide to Autogenics
https://vimeo.com/showcase/9750652

Start by getting into your preferred autogenic position.* close your eyes. Focus on the soles of your feet, move up through your ankles, calves and knees; across the thighs, the stomach and the chest allowing the shoulders to relax and moving down through the arms right to the fingertips and allow any tension to go. Now focus on the base of your spine and move slowly through your back, relaxing the muscles, moving towards the shoulders, through the neck, across the back of the head, over the head, across the forehead, eyelids and cheekbones and relax.

*See pages 8, 9 and 10 for recommended autogenic postures.

Unlike body scans that are intended as a relaxation component of other body mind practices the aim of completing a body scan before beginning your AT practice is for you to check on your body posture and comfort whilst noticing any areas of tension and sensations in and around you. As you become aware of, observe, and name each body part in turn you are quietening your body mind system in preparation for accessing the autogenic state when you start your AT practice.

Your dominant arm

Depending on whether you are left or right handed, choose the hand you use most (which is your dominant hand) and say after completing the body scan, 'my right/left arm is heavy'. This is a cue for your body mind system and becomes the signal for your brain to register that the autogenic process is beginning.

Your brain learns to recognise this cue as the beginning of your AT practice.

The cancel

This is the crucial final step of your AT practice and is about enabling you to safely leave the deeply relaxation of the Theta brainwave state and return to full consciousness. Just opening your eyes at the end of your AT practice without the cancel ritual you could find yourself dangerously disoriented. The cancel acts as a 'circuit breaker', enabling you to return fully to consciousness.

The cancel is done in three stages:

1. Clench your fingers and toes and pull your arms up sharply towards your chest
2. Take a deep breath
3. Have a good stretch with arms above your head whilst breathing out and opening your eyes

The cues of the dominant arm and the cancel = the two bookends of your practice. Your brain learns to recognise these cues as a signal to start the autogenic process (my left or right arm is heavy) and the cancel to finish (pull arms towards the chest, breathe, stretch, and open eyes) to come out of the deep Theta state.

Passive concentration or awareness

In order to start training and preparing your body mind system to access the Theta brainwave state, you have to be able to become a passive observer of yourself. Becoming a passive observer requires passive concentration, which we know may sound like a contradiction.

A way to understand how to become a passive observer of yourself is to imagine yourself as a video camera watching yourself and all you are doing with the accompanying sensations, feelings, and thoughts. Alternatively, imagining what having a helicopter view of your thoughts, movements, and sensations would be like can also give you an idea of the experience of passive awareness and observation.

You *do not* need to do anything except notice and observe. As Johannes Schulz said:

> The trainee's passive and casual attitude towards the intended functional changes is regarded as one of the most important factors of the autogenic approach.

It is this passive concentration or awareness that prepares the body mind system to relax enough to access the Theta brainwave state and to rebalance, repair, and renew without interference from your busy conscious mind (Gamma, Beta, or Alpha brainwave states).

It is whilst in the Theta brainwave state that your body mind system's own inbuilt self-regulating mechanism is enabled so that balance is restored and homeostasis can occur.

Autogenic discharges

An autogenic discharge sometimes occurs when we are in the autogenic state during AT practice as the border between our conscious and unconscious mind becomes more permeable. Autogenic discharges can take the form of physical sensations such as involuntary twitching of muscles or movement of limbs, numbness, feelings of pain or warmth in different parts of the body, and/or emotional responses such as crying, sighing, smiling, or laughing.

These are all natural and healthy responses to our body mind system's offloading sources of inner tension as we access our capacity for self-regulation and restore balance (homeostasis), so any repressed reactions and emotions from the effects of previous illness, injury, accident, surgical procedures, effects of any substance abuse, and/or emotional trauma can trigger an autogenic discharge.

The three autogenic training postures

To receive the most benefit from and maintain maximum responsiveness to the autogenic process and for the six AT standard exercises to have the maximum effect it is important that your body be relaxed and open without any constrictions.

The three body postures most commonly recommended and described by Johannes Schulz are illustrated and described below. We would suggest you try all three postures when you start learning AT.

The simple sitting position—SS

Sit towards the front of an upright chair without arms, with your legs comfortably apart and feet flat on the ground. The angle from knees to ground should be a little more than 90 degrees (see illustration). Get into position by straightening your spine and letting your head float upwards, whilst letting your arms hang down by your sides. Then let your hips rotate backwards and your body slouch a little in the vertical plane, relaxing your back and neck and letting your head come gently forward. Finally, place your hands comfortably on your thighs

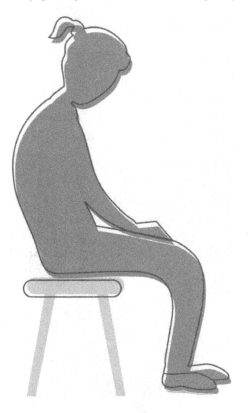

The armchair position—AP

Sit well back in a comfortable armchair so that your spine is fully supported. Lean your head against the chair back, on a cushion, or allow it to be comfortably upright in a neutral position. Your legs should be supported by the chair seat in this position. Your arms may rest, palms down, either on the arms of the chair or comfortably on your lap.

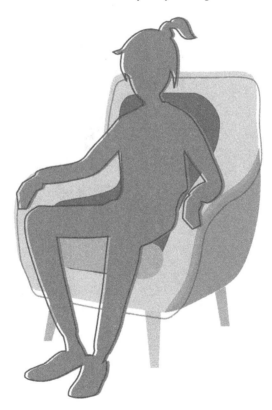

The horizontal position—HP

Lie flat with your head supported by a small cushion and, if more comfortable, with a cushion under your knees as well. Your legs should be straight with your feet slightly apart and your toes pointing outwards. Your arms rest by your sides not touching your body, with palms downwards.

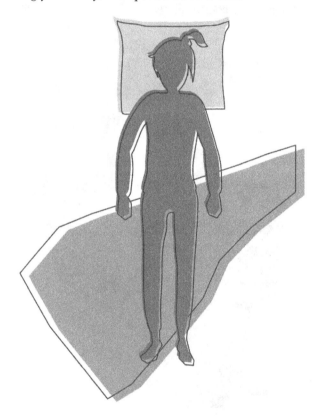

It is worth noting that although people are strongly advised to use these three postures for maintaining maximum responsiveness to the autogenic process, it has been reported by clients that even lying on their side when doing their AT practice is beneficial. So once you have learnt the six AT standard exercises, you can try other positions that you may find work just as well for you when doing your AT practice.

Always take time before you start your practice to make sure you are comfortable.

Before beginning your AT practice, it is important to remind yourself of the following aspects of your internal and external awareness that can ensure that your AT practice is successful and satisfying:

1. Make sure you are In a comfortable position in a quiet environment
2. With each of the six AT standard exercises make mental contact with the relevant part of your body
3. Be able to bring your passive awareness to any sensations arising in your body
4. Remind yourself of the importance of continuous repetition of the six AT standard exercises in multiples of three (3, 6, 9, 12, etc.). As with any associative learning with repetition, we strengthen the connection between the formulae and the psycho-physiological response. Repetitions of three are also likely linked to Johannes Schulz's practice as a hypnotist.

The six AT standard exercises build one upon another. Each of the six exercise sequences has the sole purpose of inducing and maintaining in your body mind system the autogenic state of deep relaxation (Theta brainwave state) in order to optimise your capacity for self-regulation, promote resilience, and maintain wellbeing in the various parts of your central nervous system (CNS) and your autonomous nervous system (ANS).

1. Position for all exercises is SS, AP, or HP
2. Be comfortable and make a body scan
3. Allow your awareness to focus, in a passive way, on your dominant hand and arm
4. Repeat the AT formulae/exercises silently in your mind

On the following pages, along with the instructions for each of the six standard exercises, we offer our understanding of the *rationale* behind each exercise, possible *autogenic discharges* associated with each exercise, as well as *contraindications*, i.e. when it is inadvisable to learn an exercise unless under the supervision of a qualified AT practitioner.

Johannes Schulz designed the six AT standard exercises as a do-it-yourself toolkit for use without the need for input from professional helpers, but during the learning stage you may find it helpful to have access to audio and visual prompts from an experienced AT trainer. We have therefore produced a set of short audio and video clips for each of the six AT standard exercises so you can see how to 'get it right'.

Access to these audio and video resources is via:
Introduction: Essential preparation for Autogenics
https://vimeo.com/showcase/9750652

It is important to emphasise, however, that the greatest benefits from the six AT standard exercises come from you internalising the exercises so you can repeat them silently to yourself whenever and wherever you feel the need to reconnect with and activate your body mind system's inbuilt capacity for self-regulation.

So remember the Chinese proverb:

> *I hear and I forget*
> *I see and I remember*
> *I do and I understand*

Wishing you happy and healthy learning.

First Standard Exercise Heaviness

'My arms and legs are heavy'

Rationale

Feelings of heaviness are associated with muscular relaxation as well as resting and recovery from exertion or illness and directly link with Johannes Schulz's observations in both everyday life and empirical studies of the bodily changes his patients experienced during sleep and hypnosis.

The heaviness exercises were developed following research that suggested concentrating on heaviness can enable the body mind system's relaxation response, thus activating the parasympathetic nervous system (PSNS) functions for repair, rest, recovery, and recuperation.

Schulz wanted to enable people *without* the aid of a therapist to be able to access via the relaxation response their innate capacity for self-regulation. Muscular relaxation is recognised as the first step to relieving tension and inducing a relaxation response thus the first standard exercise is about heaviness.

Possible autogenic discharges

- Intrusive thoughts
- Restlessness in limbs
- Anxiety or fear whilst doing the exercise
- Some disagreeable tingling or pulsating sensations in the fingers

Contraindications

- Dizziness or pain whilst doing the exercise
- Anyone diagnosed with a psychotic illness should not do the exercise
- Anyone with a head injury, suffering from epilepsy, or with a history of alcoholism who experiences uncomfortably strong autogenic discharges

Practice

'My arms and legs are heavy'

Week 1—days 1, 2, and 3

1. *Close your eyes—body scan*
2. *My right/left arm is heavy x 1*
3. *My right arm is heavy x 3*
4. *My left arm is heavy x 3*
5. *Both arms are heavy x 3*
6. *Cancel*

Repeat this whole exercise twice more, cancelling in between each repetition. Aim to do three sessions every day if possible—morning, midday, and evening. After practising this exercise for two more days (Days 2 and 3), add to the exercise by including your legs as follows.

Week 1—days 4, 5, 6, and 7

1. *Close your eyes—body scan*
2. *My right/left arm is heavy x 1*
3. *My right arm is heavy x 3*
4. *My left arm is heavy x 3*
5. *Both arms are heavy x 3*
6. *My right leg is heavy x 3*
7. *My left leg is heavy x 3*
8. *Both legs are heavy x 3*
9. *My arms and legs are heavy x 3*
10. *Cancel*

Repeat this whole exercise twice more, cancelling in between each repetition.

Exercise 1: Heaviness
https://vimeo.com/showcase/9750652

First Standard Exercise (Part 2)
Heaviness + Neck and Shoulders

'My neck and shoulders are heavy'

Rationale

In Week 2, in order to allow the brain time to reliably establish the new neural pathways of the relaxation response, and for the body to start releasing any stress or toxic emotions you are holding in your body mind system, you need to repeat the heaviness exercise with the addition of your neck and shoulders.

The phrases 'they get my back up' and 'they are a pain in the neck' sum up what is at the heart of the rationale of this addition to the heaviness exercise learnt in Week 1. One of the most important sources of tension in the body is from the trapezius muscles (see drawing on page 19), which cover the upper back, the back of the neck and the shoulders. Because the trapezius muscles help our heads, necks, arms, shoulders, and torsos move, it is vital they are as relaxed as possible.

The drawing on page 19 shows how the trapezius muscles extend in a diamond shape from the nape of the neck across the shoulders and down the back to a central point midway down the spine. Nowadays, when many of us spend long periods of time hunched over a keyboard, tension builds in our neck and shoulders, then transfers to our trapezius muscles and impacting on our backs. Many osteopaths and medical professionals recognise that chronic back and hip pain can be attributed to stress which is held in the neck and shoulders.

Tension headaches can be caused by contraction of muscles at the back of the neck or tension knots in the neck and shoulder area. This is often indicative of more general stress in your body mind system and is a common area in which many people experience tension. Anger can also cause tension hence the two phrases mentioned earlier.

Directing your passive concentration and awareness to heaviness in the neck and shoulders can help reduce tension and ease any stress symptoms in these areas of your body.

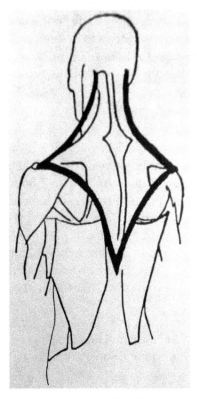

Trapezius Muscle

Possible autogenic discharges

- Tremors—involuntary shaking/twitching in the upper body or shoulders
- Sudden twinges or pain in shoulders or upper back

Contraindications

If you have had neck or shoulder surgery or injury recently, please check with your GP or physio before adding in the neck and shoulder exercise.

In Week 2, we also include an additional phrase which is inserted after you say my neck and shoulders are heavy at the end of each exercise sequence and before you go into the cancel. You can either use the phrase '*I am at peace*' or alternatively '*I am relaxed*'. This is the only formula which is not linked to a bodily function.

Rationale

The rationale for including this phrase is that it gives you the opportunity to extend the calm you are hopefully beginning to feel, thus keeping you in the Theta brainwave state for a longer time. The statement '*I am at peace*' or '*I am relaxed*' can also help you maintain a feeling of positivity as even if you are not feeling relaxed or at peace your intention is likely to be to attain such a state of calm. So adding in this phrase is in part motivational and in part aspirational of a state you wish to attain.

Once you have learnt the six AT standard exercises, you may want to add in other motivational and personal formulae or phrases, and you will find some examples on page 39, where we describe Week 8.

Practice

'My neck and shoulders are heavy'

Week 2—Days 1, 2, 3, 4, 5, 6, and 7

1. Close your eyes—body scan
2. My right/left arm is heavy x 1
3. My arms and legs are heavy x 3
4. My neck and shoulders are heavy x 3
5. I am relaxed or I am at peace x 3
6. Cancel

The partial exercise

During Week 2 practice, use *'my neck and shoulders are heavy'* as a partial exercise so that you frequently repeat the phrase to yourself throughout the day wherever you are.

Saying *'my neck and shoulders are heavy'* can be used as a partial exercise in between your regular daily practise of the six AT standard exercises. This partial exercise can be carried out with your eyes wide open, and you don't need to use one of the AT postures. All you need to do is silently repeat to yourself *'my neck and shoulders are heavy'* over and over again in bursts of 3, 9, 12, 15, and so on repetitions.

Because of the new neural pathways you are establishing, use *'my neck and shoulders are heavy'* as a partial exercise in the midst of daily life can become a quick way of relieving stress and tension and reconnecting with the Theta brainwave state induced by the relaxation response produced when doing your AT practice.

When practising *'my neck and shoulders are heavy'*, picture in your mind the trapezius muscles, as seen in the drawing on page XX, so that you can focus your passive awareness on your neck and shoulders.

This can be done numerous times per day and has been shown to be hugely helpful in maintaining relaxed shoulders, neck, and hence a more relaxed *you*!

As you continue practising the heaviness exercise, you may also feel warmth in various parts of your body. This feeling of warmth provides a natural segue into Week 3 and the second standard AT exercise—warmth.

Exercise 2: Neck and shoulders
https://vimeo.com/showcase/9750652

Second Standard Exercise Warmth

'My arms and legs are warm'

Rationale

Feelings of warmth are associated with increased blood flow to the skin, so the warmth exercise was originally developed as a result of two observations Schultz made. First, he observed how the effect on agitated patients of warm baths helped create feelings of calmness and relaxation. Second, he observed that patients undergoing hypnosis reported initially experiencing feelings of heaviness, which were then followed by feelings of warmth.

Schulz and Luthe later (1969) found by comparing the effectiveness of the six AT standard exercises in relieving symptoms that 50% of all improvements took place during the second and fifth exercises, the two warmth-related exercises.

Possible autogenic discharges

- Involuntary movements
- Trembling
- Salivation
- Increased feelings of warmth
- Increased feeling of heaviness in the body

Contraindications

The warmth exercises affect our circulatory system, so this exercise can be difficult for people who have poor circulation. Anyone suffering from acrocyanosis (a condition where small blood vessels constrict, leading to a decrease in blood flow and oxygen moving to your extremities, causing the skin to turn blue) may have difficulty in achieving warmth. If this is the case for you, please concentrate on these two formulae for no longer than two minutes.

When the warmth formula elicits strong reactions in the circulatory system, e.g. vasoconstriction (when blood vessels constrict so blood flow is reduced, which may raise blood pressure) or vasodilation (widening of blood vessels so there is an increase in blood flowing through arteries which can cause lowering of blood pressure—hypotension) consult a qualified AT practitioner.

Many people with poor circulation choose to repeat Week 3—second standard exercise—several times, practising the heaviness and warmth for one or two more weeks before moving on to the next standard exercise, as experience shows the feeling of warmth can increase with regular practise.

Of course, when the outside temperature is very high it might be uncomfortable to do the warmth exercises.

Practice

'My arms and legs are warm'

Week 3—Days 1, 2, 3, 4, 5, 6, and 7:
warmth in arms and legs

1. *Close your eyes—body scan*
2. *My right/left arm is heavy X 1*
3. *My arms and legs are heavy x 3*
4. *(Continuing with dominant arm first)*
5. *My right/left arm is warm x 3*
6. *My left/right arm is warm x 3*
7. *Both arms are warm x 3*
8. *My right/left leg is warm x 3*
9. *My left/right leg is warm x 3*
10. *Both legs are warm x 3*
11. *My arms and legs are warm x 3*
12. *My neck and shoulders are heavy x 3*
13. *I am at peace/relaxed x 3*
14. *Cancel*

Exercise 3: Warmth
https://vimeo.com/showcase/9750652

Third Standard Exercise Cardiac Regulation

'My heartbeat is calm and regular'

Rationale

Whilst there are times when we are aware of our heartbeat and pulse, mostly these natural rhythms in our body carry on 24/7 outside of our awareness. During the heaviness and warmth exercises, people often report becoming aware of their heart beating, and Schulz and Luthe's research showed that their patients' cardiac function could slow down during heaviness and warmth exercises.

We now also know heart rate variability (HRV) is one indicator of wellbeing and resilience. So the third standard exercise formula: *'my heartbeat is calm and regular'* is designed to support cardiac self-regulation, the slowing of our heart rate and lowering of our blood pressure.

If you have noticed whilst practising your AT standard exercises 1 and 2 that your heart rate seems to have slowed down, this can be viewed as an indication of your accessing the deep relaxation state. This third exercise is designed to help and reinforce the positive effects standard exercises 1 and 2 may have had on your cardiac regulation.

Before you start this new exercise, try and locate your heart by putting a hand on your chest where you think your heart is and allow yourself to feel the heartbeat by placing your fingertips over the area. Create an awareness of your heartbeat and be able to mentally tune in to where it is.

However, whilst it can be useful for your passive concentration to focus on the location of your heart in your body, there is no need to try and influence your heartbeat. Just observe passively what happens when you say, *'my heartbeat is calm and regular'*.

Possible autogenic discharges

- Faster heartbeat
- Pressure in chest
- Faster breathing
- Slower breathing
- Pulsating sensations

Contraindications

Do not continue with the exercise if you experience tension or an increase in tension anywhere in your body, if you have extreme anxiety about your heart and/or experience your heart beating rapidly when doing this exercise, or if suffering from hyperthyroidism (over active thyroid), which can cause rapid or irregular heartbeat should not do this exercise.

Practice

'My heartbeat is calm and regular'

Week 4—Days 1, 2, 3, 4, 5, 6, and 7

1. *Close your eyes—body scan*
2. *My right/left arm is heavy x 1*
3. *My arms and legs are heavy and warm x 3*
4. *My heartbeat is calm and regular x 3*
5. *My neck and shoulders are heavy x 3*
6. *I am at peace/relaxed x 3*
7. *Cancel*

Exercise 4: Heartbeat
https://vimeo.com/showcase/9750652

Fourth Standard Exercise Respiration

'My body breathes for me'

Rationale

This exercise focuses on slower deeper breathing and reduction in oxygen consumption. It is important during this exercise that you focus on the bridge of your nose and not on your lungs, as this allows uninterrupted rebalancing of your breathing by your body mind system. This is generally a very relaxing formula and usually leads to a deepening of your relaxation response as well as of feelings of warmth, and heaviness. You should become aware that your response to any physical and emotional stress also improves.

The phrase we recommend *'my body breathes for me'* is adapted from the original German formula *'es atmet mich'*, which translates as *it breathes me* as the 'ES' in German refers to *das korper* = the body being a neuter word, and so the literal translation is *it breathes me*.

If you look at the phrases *'it breathes me'* or *'my body breathes for me'*, you will see how both formulae allow you to simply passively observe your breathing without your needing to or trying to take control.

In fact, breathing as an ANS function happens automatically and is most of the time out of our control. So by simply passively observing your breathing, you give your body mind system permission to self-regulate and rebalance. As you stay in the position of being a passive observer, you allow your body to moderate your breathing.

The first three standard exercises will hopefully have had a positive influence on your respiration and will have resulted in slower and deeper breathing. You may yourself have noticed such a change by this stage. The breathing formulae is designed to reinforce any such changes by passively focussing your attention on your breath response.

The key to this exercise is to let go of all attempts at controlled breathing responses and allow the breathing to occur as naturally as possible.

Possible autogenic discharges

It is quite rare to experience intense or disagreeable autogenic discharges during this exercise.

Discharges most often reported as occurring during this exercise are:

- Faster breathing
- Breathing more relaxed and slower
- Increased involuntary movements, such as twitches in the body, arms, and or legs
- Concentration easier
- Feelings of warmth in the cardiac region

Contraindications

Do not do the respiration exercise if you have a functional disorder of the respiratory system or asthma or tuberculosis.

From now on, you do not need to cancel between each repetition of the exercise sequence, but you can flow through from one repetition to the other.

If doing the exercises before going to sleep or if you should wake up during the night, no cancelling is required at all, so you can just keep repeating the exercise and then gently fall back to sleep.

Practice

'My body breathes for me'

Week 5—Days 1, 2, 3, 4, 5, 6, and 7

1. *Close your eyes—body scan*
2. *My right/left arm is heavy x 1*
3. *My arms and legs are heavy and warm x 3*
4. *My heartbeat is calm and regular x 3*
5. *My body breathes for me x 3*
6. *My neck and shoulders are heavy x 3*
7. *I am at peace/relaxed x 3*
8. *Cancel*

Exercise 5: Breath
https://vimeo.com/showcase/9750652

Fifth Standard Exercise
Abdominal Warmth

'My solar plexus is warm'

Rationale

In everyday language, we often say, 'I am sick to my stomach' or 'that gives me butterflies in my stomach'. This is the sympathetic nervous system (SNS) responding to fear or anxiety and both sensations originate in the solar plexus. This exercise can restore homeostasis in the gut and other abdominal organs.

The solar plexus situated behind the stomach is a complex system of radiating nerves and ganglia that govern the autonomic nervous system (ANS). A spaghetti-like junction, it plays an important role in the functioning of our stomach, kidneys, liver, and adrenal glands.

As always, when starting a new AT exercise, it is most important to be mentally in contact with the area of the body to which we are bringing our passive concentration. The solar plexus can be a challenge for some people as it is not an organ and is also not something we generally talk about on a daily basis.

One good way of locating the solar plexus is to imagine drawing a line vertically from top to bottom through your body as if cutting it in half vertically and then drawing a line horizontally midway across your body. Where the two lines meet is roughly where your solar plexus (SP) is located.

Applying warmth to the abdominal area is known to have positive effects. For instance, people will often use a hot water bottle applied to their stomach to comfort and calm down a stomach ache. When the warmth of the hot water bottle is applied, the nervous system becomes calmer as your muscles relax. Sometimes people can even experience feelings of drowsiness.

The use of the formula *'my solar plexus is warm'* is intended to induce these warm feelings.

Possible autogenic discharges

You might experience some of the following sensations—all mostly pleasant:

- Prickling in the abdomen
- Some tummy rumbling
- Feelings of pulsating
- Salivation
- Falling asleep

During this exercise, there can also be increased motor discharges, such as feeling the need to cry or electrical-like sensations, which usually pass quite quickly and are often related to experiences in your past held in cell memory, e.g. wounds, injuries, and damage that your body has had to work to repair.

Contraindications

If you have digestive tract problems, such as acute gastritis, stomach ulcers, or acid in your stomach, then leave this formula out. If you are or think you might be pregnant, do not use this exercise. If whilst doing this exercise you suddenly experience abdominal pain, don't continue with this exercise.

Practice

'My solar plexus is warm'

Week 6—Days 1, 2, 3, 4, 5, 6, and 7

1. *Close your eyes—body scan*
2. *My right/left arm is heavy x 1*
3. *My arms and legs are heavy and warm x 3*
4. *My heartbeat is calm and regular x 3*
5. *My body breathes for me x 3*
6. *My solar plexus is warm x 3*
7. *My neck and shoulders are heavy x 3*
8. *I am at peace/relaxed x 3*
9. *Cancel*

Exercise 6: Solar plexus
https://vimeo.com/showcase/9750652

Sixth Standard Exercise Cooling of the Forehead

'My forehead is cool and clear'

Rationale

Schultz observed how in addition to the soothing effects of warm baths on his patients, a cold compress placed on their foreheads induced an even greater sense of calm.

Just as we often say, 'I need to clear my head' or 'they have a very clear head', it seems that the coolness of the forehead creates a relaxed alertness in contrast to the warmth of the warmth-inducing exercises that can lead to feelings of drowsiness and deep relaxation. So Schulz and Luthe added the sixth standard exercise inducing a state of mental calm and a clear head to complete the sequence of the six AT standard exercises.

As with all the other formulae, you need to bring your attention and focus to your forehead. You are *not*, however, trying to make your forehead cool—just say the words silently interiorly and passively observe your forehead in your mind.

Whilst doing this exercise, you may experience a mild feeling of coolness or sometimes even a gentle breath effect around your forehead, rather like the draft from a window. It is unlikely that any strong reactions are experienced with this exercise.

Possible autogenic discharges

- Feeling cooler
- Twitching of muscles is sometimes notable in the anal area

Contraindications

Not suitable for people who have suffered or are suffering from a brain injury or epilepsy. Not to be used if you suffer from migraines or the exercise activates a headache.

Practice

'My forehead is cool and clear'

Week 7—Days 1, 2, 3, 4, 5, 6, and 7

1. *Close your eyes—body scan*
2. *My right/left arm is heavy x 1*
3. *My arms and legs are heavy and warm x 3*
4. *My heartbeat is calm and regular x 3*
5. *My body breathes for me x 3*
6. *My solar plexus is warm x 3*
7. *My forehead is cool and clear x 3*
8. *My neck and shoulders are heavy x 3*
    1.
9. *I am at peace/relaxed x 3*
    2.
10. *Cancel*
    3.

Exercise 7: Forehead
https://vimeo.com/showcase/9750652

The complete sequence of six AT standard exercises

Rationale

Week 8 may look like a repeat of Week 7, but this repetition of the complete sequence of six AT standard exercises without introducing anything new is needed to further embed the learning of the sequences in our neural pathways.

We know repetition creates habits, and AT is a habit that is good for our health!

For some people, adding personal motivational and intentional formulae into their AT practice after saying, '*my neck and shoulders are heavy*' can be extremely beneficial if a particular behavioural change is wanted. Some examples would be 'I allow myself to succeed'; 'I eat only enough'; 'I am calm about lecturing'; formulae should be short, simple, in the present tense, and be a positive statement about something you want to achieve and/or something you long to be. So statements might state with 'I expect …' or 'I am managing …' or 'I am choosing …' Motivational and intentional formulae work on the same principle as autosuggestion.

Practice

Week 8—Days 1, 2, 3, 4, 5, 6, and 7

1. *Close your eyes—body scan*
2. *My right/left arm is heavy x 1*
3. *My arms and legs are heavy and warm x 3*
4. *My heartbeat is calm and regular x 3*
5. *My body breathes for me x 3*
6. *My solar plexus is warm x 3*
7. *My forehead is cool and clear x 3*
8. *My neck and shoulders are heavy x 3*
9. *I am at peace/relaxed x 3*
10. *Cancel*

Exercise 8: Complete exercise sequence
https://vimeo.com/showcase/9750652

You have now learnt all six AT standard exercises, and we hope that practising them using the instructions in the above pages, maybe accompanied by the audio and video clips, has shown you the effectiveness of the exercises and whetted your appetite for including the six standard exercises as part of your daily self-care routine.

PART 2

BACKGROUND INFORMATION

WHY NOW?

Present times (the 2020s) are challenging for so many of us in a century that has already seen an increase in collective and individual trauma worldwide. Stress for many has become an unavoidable part of our 21st-century lives. But whilst we may not be able to avoid life's pressures, we can change the way we respond to stressors by supporting our resilience and our body mind's own capacity for self-regulation and balance. In our digital age, many of us now have unprecedented almost immediate exposure via the media to the consequences of traumatic world events.

A small sample from the first two decades of the 21st century of some of the causes of disease, death, financial and physical hardship, poverty, and displacement of populations due to terrorist activity would be 9/11, tsunamis (2004 Asia) and hurricanes (2005 Katrina), financial crisis (2008), political uprisings and protests (Arab spring 2011), earthquakes (NZ 2011), and in 2022 the turmoil unknown since Second World War caused by the Russian invasion of Ukraine.

Whether we live through these events ourselves, see and hear about them via TV, radio, or social media or know people in our personal or professional lives who are caught up in one or other of the traumatic events regularly occurring, both our resilience and capacity for adaptation are constantly being tested.

Beginning at the end of 2019, the worldwide impact of the pandemic proved to be a shocking challenge for us all as the health and economic effects rippled out across the world. Those of us in the Western world privileged enough to have enough to eat, places to sleep, and live in relatively safe environments had never before had our resilience tested like, for example, our parents and grandparents who were alive during the Second World War. But the ongoing uncertainty from the threat of Russian expansionism, the need to attend to the millions of displaced persons needing refuge in today's world, as well as the distress due to the inequalities caused by the gap between rich and poor are now playing havoc with our autonomic nervous systems.

We are in unfamiliar territory as the virus named COVID-19 constantly presents us with real threats, thus activating our sympathetic nervous system (SNS). We already know that when we are fearful and on high alert over prolonged periods of time, navigating life's challenges can for some generate symptoms of stress and distress: anxiety, insomnia, palpitations, fatigue, depression, etc. all of which deplete our resilience and compromise our immune system.

It would not be an exaggeration to say that most of us, whether we know it or not, whether we have symptoms or not, have been living in a heightened state of arousal, that is, with our sympathetic nervous system dominant at least since the onset of the pandemic in 2020. Now, as we write in 2022, there is no indication that this will change any time soon. So it is all the more important that as individuals we understand that we can access our body mind system's innate capacity for self-regulation as an aid to supporting our immune system and maintaining our resilience.

WHAT FOR?

Learning AT gives a person a permanent portable skillset that can be learnt and used with or without the help of an AT practitioner. The six AT standard exercises once learnt are economic of time and thus a good fit for busy people. In our digital age, more and more people recognise the importance of having a repertoire of tools for self-care and self-empowerment in daily life.

It was the original vision of Johannes Schulz, the creator of AT, that the six AT standard exercises would provide a self-help tool that people could learn and use without the need for the involvement of a healthcare professional. With the demands of today's world, we need to pay attention to our 'bank balance' of resilience and to strengthening and supporting our immune system.

Just as we check that our computer systems are regularly updated, staying abreast of new IT developments so they can function optimally, so we need to do the same with the resources we have in our repertoire of health maintenance and disease prevention 'operating systems'—the self-care tools we have for our body mind system.

Our aim with this book is to make available to people the possibility of easily learning AT—because we are convinced that, as a self-care skillset, it offers substantial health benefits to cope with and navigate today's world.

We know that when we are stressed and in a state of hyper-arousal or hypoarousal our resilience can be compromised and our immune system weakened, so a tool like AT that can restore the balance between our sympathetic (SNS) and para-sympathetic (PSNS) nervous systems eliciting the relaxation response is for us an invaluable resource for self-care.

WHO FOR?

AT is about health maintenance and disease prevention, so any-one appreciating the connection between our body mind system and our general wellbeing will find AT both interesting and beneficial. AT as described in this book is intended as a resource for you if you want to take charge as much as possible of build-ing up and protecting your own wellbeing and resilience.

Regular use of the six AT standard exercises provides us with a skillset designed for health promotion and strengthen-ing our immune system. By enabling us to access the relaxation response (first described by Herbert Benson in 1975), we can ensure better overall mental and physical health and wellbeing both now and in the future.

Whilst AT is not offered as a replacement for conventional medicine, in some circumstances people do report finding AT is their preferred and effective alternative to taking medication for stress-related symptoms like insomnia, anxiety, etc.

AT is also for those who are willing to set aside some time to learn a set of new tools that will benefit their overall physical and mental health. Learning the six AT standard exercises requires an initial commitment of approximately 12 hours for the eight lessons and an ongoing commitment to three times daily practise of fewer than ten minutes.

Times of living with chronic uncertainty can lead to potentially dangerous states of hyperarousal or hypoarousal, with our body mind systems continuously on high alert. AT therefore provides an ideal self-care tool for physical and emotional self-regulation.

Many of our clients report almost immediate symptom relief or disappearance once they have learnt the six AT standard exercises. This is especially important in today's world of shrinking resources as people with symptoms that are not life-threatening probably have very limited or no access to health professionals' expertise, despite, for example, suffering the stress-induced consequences due to prolonged periods of lockdown.

The six AT standard exercises can be safely learnt by most people from age 15 years and upwards, except when there is a severe mental health issue together with symptoms of psychosis; or if there are ongoing cardiac problems.

There is more detail about health conditions for which practising AT is not advised in the section called contraindications included with the description of each of the six AT standard exercises in Part 1 of this book. Whilst people with any of the conditions we list can learn the six AT standard exercises, they should arrange to be taught by a qualified AT practitioner who can monitor and adapt the pace of their learning as necessary depending on a person's responses and feedback as they are learning the six AT standard exercises.

There is reliable evidence that children too can learn AT with the help of parents and/or other adults, along with supervision by an experienced AT practitioner.

WHAT IS AT?

The six AT standard exercises are a series of mental exercises that can be self-taught, or learnt with a qualified AT practitioner, that enable us to quickly and efficiently access our body mind system's capacity for self-regulation ... the 'autogenic state'.

Johannes Schulz described the 'autogenic state' as a body mind state which brings about a psycho-physiological shift that activates the parasympathetic nervous system (PSNS). It is the PSNS mechanisms for rest, repair and restoration that quietens the fight, flight and freeze mechanisms of the sympathetic nervous system (SNS), thus enabling our body mind system's inbuilt capacity for self-regulation to bring us to a state of balance (homeostasis).

These two systems, SNS and PSNS, together with the ENS, make up our autonomic nervous system ANS and are designed to work together, helping regulate and maintain a healthy body mind system balance (homeostasis) for us.

Understanding the wonderfully delicate attunement between the parts of our central nervous system (CNS) and our autonomic nervous system (ANS) is crucial to appreciating both what AT is and how AT works. The infographic/illustration on the next page shows how our ANS is part of our central nervous system (CNS).

Our brain controls everything that is going on in our body in order to make sure all systems are operating well and it is by means of an intricate system of nerve cells (neuroreceptors) that our brain receives information about how our body is functioning. This control centre is called the central nervous system (CNS), which consists of the spinal column and the brain. We then find other nerves radiating off the spinal column to all parts of the body and this is known as the peripheral nervous system (PNS)

The vagus or wandering nerve shown on the diagram is the longest nerve of the ANS and serves as the body mind system's super highway, carrying information between the brain and the internal organs. Operating below the level of our conscious minds, the vagus nerve is an essential part of the parasympathetic nervous system (PSNS) and vital for keeping our bodies healthy. Vagal tone or the strength of our vagus nerve response naturally varies from person to person. So people with stronger vagal tone are able to relax and repair faster after encountering stressors. Conversely, low vagal tone is associated with chronic inflammation that if persistent can damage our vital organs. Along with activities like gargling, singing, belly breathing, humming, chanting, etc., the six AT standard exercises activate our capacity for self-regulation whilst simultaneously strengthening our vagus nerve and increasing vagal tone … health and wellbeing.

The central nervous system (CNS) is divided into the autonomic nervous system (ANS) and the somatic nervous system (SNS). Any dysfunction in either the ANS or SNS will negatively impact on other parts of our body mind system. Our SNS has motor pathways as well as sensory pathways, which control movement and muscles throughout the body. Our ANS only has motor pathways and controls, mainly out of our conscious awareness, our bodily functions, such as heartbeat, breathing, digestion, fight-or-flight responses, etc.

The ANS is made up of two subsystems: the sympathetic nervous system (SNS) and the parasympathetic nervous system (PSNS). One acts as an accelerator and the other as a brake. The SNS is the accelerator and helps our body activate responses to actual or perceived threat, stressful or traumatic situations with fight, flight, or freeze responses. The PSNS works like a brake and moderates our body's response to stress by helping the self-regulation process through rest, recovery, digestion and relaxation, calming heart rate, etc.

It is when these two systems (the SNS and PSNS) are working in tandem that our inbuilt capacity for self-regulation can maintain a healthy body mind system balance for us.

Everyday life in the 21st century can be stressful, causing many temporary imbalances in our body mind system, which in response produces increased levels of the hormones cortisol or adrenalin. Over time high levels of either hormone can trigger nutrient deficiencies that in turn adversely affect our digestion leading to cell damage and/or inflammation. Cell damage or inflammation means our neurotransmitters are not being released correctly, so symptoms of stress, such as anxiety, depression, difficulty sleeping, etc., then appear.

Clearly, it is vital our ANS functions well and remains as well-balanced as possible. Regular AT practice neutralises the effects of too much cortisol and adrenalin in our body mind system, reducing 'brain fog' or 'body fog' so we can then think and function better.

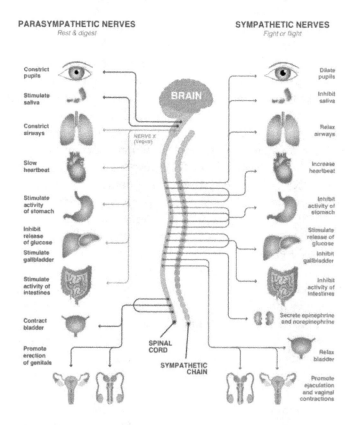

HOW DOES AT WORK?

Johannes Schulz and Wolfgang Luthe co-authored the book *Autogenic Methods* (1959), which was based on Schulz's first book published in 1932, with its subsequent updates all only available in German. *Autogenic Methods* describes in English how AT works:

> From the technical point of view, the autogenic approach hinges initially on bringing about a psycho-physiological shift (Umschaltung) from a normal state to the autogenic state which facilitates and mobilises the otherwise inhibited activity of recuperative and self-normalising brain mechanisms. The shift to the autogenic state is facilitated by conditions involving a significant reduction in afferent and efferent impulses, and the regular practise of short periods of passive concentration upon psychologically adapted stimuli (i.e. the autogenic standard formulae).

Schulz and Luthe say about passive concentration:

> The trainee's passive and casual attitude towards the intended functional changes is regarded as one of the most important factors of the autogenic approach.
>
> *(These quotes are literal translations into English from the original written by Schulz and Luthe in German)*

With the development of brainwave research in the 20th century, we now know that the *'psycho-physiological shift'* that Luthe and Schulz describe above most likely occurs when we access the relaxation response and enter the Theta brainwave state. It is when in the Theta brainwave state that our body mind system's inbuilt capacity for self-regulation and the restoration of balance between the SNS and PSNS and ENS is optimised.

The six AT standard exercises enable us to efficiently and reliably access the Theta brainwave state—the brainwave state that allows our body mind system to reboot and relax so reducing the harmful effects of external and internal stressors and thus enabling us to function more healthily.

Regular three times daily AT practice supports our ANS as it responds to the way our body mind system reacts to the many internal (within our body) and external (from the environment) stimuli we are constantly processing whether asleep or awake.

So AT works by rebalancing our brain chemistry, neutralising the effects of increased levels of cortisol and adrenalin in our body mind system, so we can then think and function better. As we have said, our clients report that practising AT reduces the 'brain fog' or 'body fog'.

Brainwave states

As long as we are alive, our brain constantly produces different bursts of electrical activity called brainwave states as neurons and neurotransmitters communicate with one another. This electrical activity in our brains changes depending on what we are doing and how we are feeling. So, for example, when we are reading our brain waves are very different from when we are relaxing.

Brainwave states or rhythms can be measured by an EEG machine, which measures the electrical activity in the cerebral cortex. The EEG machine (first recording made in 1887) amplifies the signals from our brains and records them in a wave pattern on graph paper (electroencephalogram), which provides information about our health and state of mind.

The human brainwave diagram on the next page shows five different brainwave states, each of which operates at a different speed. From fastest to slowest, they are Gamma, Beta, Alpha, Theta, and Delta.

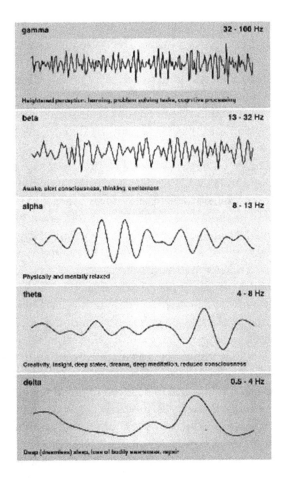

When we are focussed on finishing a difficult crossword, we are likely to be in the Gamma brainwave state, and when we finish and decide to go to bed and read for a few minutes before attempting sleep, we are then likely to be in the Beta brainwave state. When we put the book down, turn off the light, and close our eyes we go into the Alpha brainwave state. Then as we become drowsy we are in the Theta brainwave state, and finally when we fall asleep we go into the Delta brainwave state.

Gamma can be understood to be when we are in our peak concentration and problem-solving mode and when we are fully engaged in processing information, problem-solving, and learning.

Beta can be understood to be when we are busy with active minds, wide awake, alert, and focussed whilst going about our daily activities, making decisions and focussed on the external world. A person in active conversation, a debater, a teacher, or a talk show host are all in Beta when working.

Alpha can be understood to be a restful, reflective, thinking state, for example, when stretching upon waking up and maybe turning off our alarm clock. Our brain is relaxed not being asked to process a lot of information, so in a state of wakeful rest. Another example of Alpha could be when we decide to take a break from a conference and go for a walk in the garden to relax and unwind.

Importantly Alpha appears to bridge the conscious and the unconscious and is the major rhythm seen when we are relaxed, calm, and focussed on learning or doing our jobs. We can increase Alpha by closing our eyes or deep breathing or decrease Alpha by thinking or calculating. Some people associate Alpha with mindfulness.

Theta can be understood to be when we are dozing, drowsy, or daydreaming. Sometimes described as slow activity, the Theta brainwave state is seen as connected with creativity, intuition, daydreaming and fantasising, and reverie. Theta brainwaves are strong during internal focus, meditation, prayer, and spiritual awareness. Equally, motorway driving can induce the Theta state due to the repetitious nature of that form of driving. For example, when we discover we have been on 'auto pilot' and can't recall the last 5 miles of the road in contrast to driving on an unfamiliar country road where concentration (the Beta brainwave state) is required in order to drive safely. The Theta brainwave state is a state where tasks become so automatic that the conscious mind seems to disengage from the task.

The Theta brainwave state is also the state of mental relaxation associated with the flow of creativity and ideas—so, for example, we often say we had a good idea when in the shower, bath, whilst jogging, or taking a walk. Also, it is during meditation that our brains show Theta brainwaves.

Delta can be understood as our deepest level of relaxation and restorative healing sleep—a deep dreamless sleep.

In our view, it is the Theta brainwave state that most approximates to the autogenic state described by Schulze and Luthe. We make no claim to being 'right' and acknowledge that other AT practitioners equate the autogenic state with the Alpha brainwave state

What happens to us when we go into the Theta brainwave state is that we are not consciously thinking or in control of what is going on in our minds. We have literally 'switched off'. It is then that the self-regulating capacity built into our ANS can, without interference, enable our body mind system to rebalance via homeostasis

It is this state of profound relaxation accessed when practising AT that can have transformative effects on our body mind system, easily dissolving any symptoms of stress: anxiety or allied symptoms.

Once learnt, regular daily use of AT enables us quickly to access the Theta brainwave state and so rebalance and function more efficiently and effectively, as well as providing us with a powerful resource for health maintenance and disease prevention.

AT is a resource that enables us by ourselves, without depending on an external professional, to access this resource which calms us and reconnects us with our inbuilt capacity for self-regulation and balance. A balance is necessary for our resilience and for optimally managing inevitable life stressors day by day. When we practise AT, we are enabling the body mind system to return to its natural self-regulating state.

WHEN TO USE AT?

AT is most beneficial for health maintenance and reducing symptoms of stress when practised three times daily—morning, midday, and evening. The six AT standard exercises enable our body mind system to self-regulate, thus calming arousal, supporting the parasympathetic system to rest, repair, and relax and thus promoting our resilience.

We gain most from the six AT standard exercises, as with other forms of exercise that benefit our body mind system, like jogging, going to the gym, meditation, mindfulness, etc., by including our AT practice as part of our daily self-care routine.

As with other forms of exercise, AT supports our health maintenance efforts, boosts resilience, and reduces the potential for damage to our immune system due to symptoms of stress, such as anxiety, high blood pressure, insomnia, IBS, etc.

AT's unique selling point is that once learnt it is economic of time and can be practised anywhere. Making time to practise the six AT standard exercises whenever we unexpectedly find ourselves in a stressful situation or find ourselves worrying about an event we anticipate could generate stress is wise self-care and preventative medicine.

WHEN NOT TO USE AT (CONTRAINDICATIONS)

If you suffer from one or other of the physical and emotional conditions listed below, you *must* only learn AT under the supervision of a qualified AT practitioner who will ask you for a full medical history and may want to work with you in collaboration with your medical practitioner.

The conditions are: cardiac problems, diabetes, glaucoma, psychosis, severe depression, substance abuse, degenerative diseases, chronic psychosomatic illnesses, anxiety, insomnia, obsessive-compulsive disorders (OCD), agoraphobia, if you have suffered prolonged periods of unconsciousness, or suffer from the side effects of other chronic illnesses.

Modified versions of the six AT standard exercises are often taught to people suffering from any of the above conditions but *only* under the supervision of a qualified AT practitioner. AT is a simple and powerful tool which can usually be adapted to meet your needs if you are someone in search of better emotional and physical balance/homeostasis for your body mind system.

Be aware, however, that depending on your medical condition medical practitioners may sometimes advise against practising AT.

PART 3

THE HISTORY OF AUTOGENICS

People, places, dates, and ideas relevant to the development of Autogenics internationally

Autogenic Training has been around now for nearly 100 years and is practised across Canada, Europe, Japan, and Australia. During the last half of the 20th century, AT increased in popularity in the UK, USA, and Australia. Most of those pioneering the use of AT were trained by Johannes Schulz or Wolfgang Luthe in Germany or Canada between the 1960s and mid-1980s.

In this section, we list some of the people and ideas that influenced Johannes Schulz, the creator of AT, when he was a young physician during the early 1900s in Germany. We hope to show how Schulz's ideas were both of his time and, given developments in neuroscience in the last 30 years, ahead of his time. AT, as created by Johannes Schulz, like any significant scientific development, in recent years has provided opportunities for other health professionals and researchers to develop and apply AT according to their own professional interests and the health needs they have identified in their locality.

Thus there are a variety of adaptations of AT worldwide inspired by and/or linked to the practise of Autogenics in health services devoted to promoting health and wellbeing. The people, places, ideas, and dates here are by no means exhaustive.

The 'story' of Autogenics, like the history of many innovations, includes people, places, and events not in a linear order, so we try here to give a flavour of the overlapping of ideas, lives, and events from Schulz's creation of Autogenics to the present day.

Oscar Vogt (1870–1959)—German neurologist, hypnotist and brain researcher famous for creating the first map of the human frontal cortex and seen as a pioneer of modern neuroscience. Vogt researched the therapeutic use of hypnosis and was interested in the connection between the body and the mind.

His observations that some of his patients were able to create their own hypnotic trance state led to the creation of the term autohypnosis and were pivotal in Schulz's later formulation of the six AT standard exercises.

Korbiniam Brodman (1868–1918)—German neurologist famous for mapping the cerebral cortex and defining 52 distinct regions, known as Brodman areas, according to function, which was a milestone in the development of contemporary neuroscience. Brodman met Vogt when Brodman worked as an assistant in a sanatorium in Bavaria for nervous diseases, where Vogt was the director. Working together at the beginning of the 20th century in a neurobiological laboratory in Berlin, Vogt and Brodman observed that psychiatric patients they had treated with hypnosis were able with guidance to go into a state similar to a hypnotic state for a self-determined period of time. During these short exercises patients described experiencing sensations of warmth and heaviness in their limbs, which patients then claimed reduced tension, fatigue, stress, etc.

Johannes Heinrich Schultz (1884–1970)—German neurologist, psychiatrist, and hypnotherapist creator of Autogenics. Schulz studied under Vogt for several years and influenced by many of his ideas became interested in the phenomenon of autosuggestion. Schulz wanted to develop a therapeutic approach which would avoid the passivity that he believed occurs when patients are dependent on a therapist. He first presented his findings on autogenic training to the Medical Society in Berlin in 1926. Originally called the autogenic body organ exercises the exercises were renamed the six AT standard exercises in 1928. Schulz's first book *Autogenic Training* was published in German in 1932.

Wolfgang Luthe (1922–1985)—German physician and psychotherapist who brought AT to the attention of the

English-speaking world, championing AT as a psychothera-
peutic modality. Whilst a junior trainee doctor Luthe met
Schulz and impressed with his results using AT in the care of
asthmatic patients became Schulz's protégé. Their collaboration continued throughout Schulz's lifetime despite Luthe emi-
grating to Canada in the mid-1950s. Luthe's interest in how our
innate homeostatic self-regulating mechanisms regulate not
only physiological processes but also cognitive and emotional
processes and disorders led to AT being incorporated into psychosomatic medicine, clinical psychology, and psychiatry.

Schulz and Luthe's first jointly authored book *Autogenic*
Training: A Psychophysiologic Approach In Psychotherapy (1959)
was based on Schulz's 1932 book and subsequent research,
which had hitherto only been available in German. A six-
volume series entitled *Autogenic Therapy* (1969) followed, with
Schulz, before his death, co-authoring the first three books and
Luthe adding a number of his own innovations to AT in the last
three books, which he authored alone.

John Gibbons—Australian psychologist studying autosugges-
tion began AT training with Schulz in Germany in 1958 after
seeing the healing potential of AT. Back in Australia, Gibbons
in the 1970s developed the autogenic biomemory method
as well as training his daughter Helen in AT. Helen Gibbons
herself then trained as a clinical and organisational psychologist and in 2011 founded the Autogenic Training Institute of
Australia.

Hans Selye (1907–1982)—Austrian Canadian endocrinologist,
pioneered research on the effect of cortisol in the human body
and popularised the use of the word stress in connection with
human beings. Selye first wrote (1936) about General Adaptation Syndrome (GAS). Selye's theory describes the physiological changes the body goes through when encountering the
unexpected demands of perceived or real threat or danger:

alarm—fight-or-flight response; resistance—the body mind system tries to repair itself after the initial shock of the stress; exhaustion—prolonged or chronic stress leads to fatigue, burn out, collapse, decreased stress tolerance, and weakening of the immune system.

In Canada, Luthe met and worked with Hans Selye, demonstrating the stress reduction effects of the six AT standard exercises and became a member of the International Institute of Stress founded by Hans Selye in 1975.

In 1969 Luthe travelled to Japan and introduced AT to Japan at the University Medical School in Kyushu. Today, in many universities in Japan, Autogenics is an integral part of their BioFeedback training.

Klaus Thomas (1915–1992)—German doctor, psychotherapist, and priest who studied AT with Schulz in Berlin. In 1972 Thomas became director of the J. H. Schulz Institute for Psychotherapy, Autogenic Training, and Hypnosis, established in Berlin in 1965. This institute no longer exists, but autogenic training has become an integral part of all doctor training in Germany.

In 1977, at the invitation of The BioFeedback Society of America in Orlando, Florida, Luthe taught a three-day Introduction to the Methods of Autogenic Therapy. BioFeedback practitioners at the Menninger Foundation developed techniques incorporating AT that were used in combination with BioFeedback.

Herbert Benson (1935–2022)—American physician and cardiologist founder of the Mind/Body Medical Institute at Massachusetts General Hospital who pioneered body mind research focussing on stress and the relaxation response publishing The Relaxation Response in 1975. Benson's research showed that to access the relaxation response four basic components are necessary: a quiet environment, a mental device known as a mantra, a passive attitude, and a comfortable position. Recognising these are the core components of AT in the 1970s, Benson included autogenic training on the institute's list of treatments to be used for relaxation

Malcolm Carruthers (1938)—English GP who researched the relationship between stress, tension, and coronary heart disease and was interested in the study of cortisol. Wanting to understand Selye's research into cortisol, Carruthers went to Montreal, where he was introduced to Luthe who gave him volume 2 of *Autogenic Therapy: Medical Applications.* Later (in 1977), Carruthers accepted Luthe's invitation to join an AT training for doctors in Canada.

In 1982, invited by Carruthers, Luthe gave the first AT multidisciplinary training in England, with a second training following in 1983. In 1984 the British Association for Autogenic Training and Therapy (BASFATT) was established and delivered further training in England. From 1985 the Royal Homeopathic Hospital included AT as part of their integrated treatment programme.

In 1988, the International Autogenic Conference at The Maudsley Hospital took place in London. In 1994, the Swedish Society for Autogenic Therapy was founded. In 1999, BASFATT changed its name to the British Autogenic Society (BAS).

During the 1960s and 1970s, as well as teaching on psychology and psychiatry training programmes at the Universite de Montreal and McGill University, Luthe founded his own training centre near Montreal, which attracted many international students.

Luis de Rivera (1944)—Spanish psychiatrist and a pupil of Wolfgang Luthe at McGill University in the 1970s, where he specialised in psychiatry, psychotherapy, and psychoanalysis. Rivera is President of the International Society of Autogenic Training and Psychotherapy (ICAT).

Rivera edited and published *Wolfgang Luthe Introductory Workshop: Introduction to the Methods of Autogenic Training, Therapy, and Psychotherapy* (2014). Also, in 2014 in Madrid, Rivera founded the International Committee for the Coordination of Clinical Application and Teaching of Autogenic Therapy (IACT).

In 2018, the 5th World Congress of International Society of Autogenic Training and Psychotherapy (ISATAP) took place in Madrid.

Wolfgang Linden (19??)—Clinical Psychologist Professor Emeritus in Clinical and Health Psychology at the University of British Columbia. Wolfgang trained in Canada with Luthe and has authored *The Autogenic Training Method of J.H. Schultz* (4th Edition Guildford Press) and *Autogenic Training; A Clinical Guide* (1990).

In 2022 these are some of the places where Autogenics is taught:

> Canada—The Canadian Autogenic Society (CAS) was recently established as a professional and educational organisation for autogenic practitioners and trainers in Canada. Most of their members are practising hypnotherapists or certified autogenic practitioners and/or trainers.
>
> France—Autogenics is linked to the teaching of Bio-Feedback and is seen as a psycho-physiological way of addressing the emotional impact of medical issues.
>
> Hungary—Autogenics is taught and practised by members of the Association of Relaxation and Symboltherapy.
>
> Italy—The six AT standard exercises are seen as interventions for regaining balance, wellbeing and calm, so AT is mainly used to improve emotional management and in the treatment of psychosomatic disorders induced by stress. Autogenics is also used in the field of sport in Italy to improve an athlete's approach to performance.

Spain—Autogenics is offered as a degree course with three different levels of training. Luis de Rivera has published (2014) *The Evolution of Autogenic Psychotherapy in Spain*.

We have given a short overview and recognise we do not do justice here to the many other people who and places where throughout the world autogenic training is seen as a useful therapeutic intervention.

PART 4

CASE STUDIES

There is now much evidence that AT can contribute to healing in a significant number of stress-related disorders and medical conditions. In this section, you will find four case studies of people suffering from everyday medical conditions where AT has been helpful in symptom relief: with sufferers, in addition to reporting a reduction in symptoms, saying they have become calmer, more focussed, and less stressed. We also give examples of some common diseases encountered by medical practitioners, whose patients have benefitted from the use of AT either as a stand-alone treatment intervention or alongside other treatments. At the end of this section, you will find an example of the kind of medical questionnaire all qualified AT practitioners complete with their clients before commencing AT training.

With all four case studies, clients have given permission for us to share information about their condition and treatment. In each case, clients first worked with a qualified AT practitioner who with the client could plan the pace of learning the six AT standard exercises to suit the client's needs, monitor the client's responses week by week, and make any adaptations as necessary. Once the clients had learnt the complete sequence of six AT standard exercises and felt confident to continue AT practice without the help of their AT practitioner, this was of course encouraged. All clients had the assurance that if at any time they felt it could be helpful, they could arrange a consultation with their AT practitioner.

To ensure clients' privacy, all names have been changed in the descriptions that follow.

Case study 1—pain management

Noor, age 57, was referred for AT by her orthopaedic consultant. Following a complex knee operation, she was in need of help with chronic pain in the knee area as she was not responding well to medication.

Given Noor's extreme discomfort from the knee pain, the AT practitioner fast-tracked the first four weeks of AT lessons into two weeks, and Noor was able to experience accessing the autogenic state. Whilst in the autogenic state, and with the AT practitioner's help, Noor could then focus on her knee. The AT practitioner offered Noor a few different ways for her to mentally focus on the knee to try to mentally reduce the pain whilst in an autogenic state. The phrase Noor found most helpful and produced the best body mind responses was: 'my knee is cool and healing'. Using this phrase, known by AT practitioners as an 'organ-specific formula', whilst still in the autogenic state at the end of her AT practice and before the cancel seemed to help Noor's pain reduce.

Noor completed learning the six AT standard exercises using the phrase 'my knee is cool and healing'. Over the course of three months, her pain gradually decreased, and she was also able to stop taking all medication.

It is well known that non-pharmacological interventions aimed at modifying factors that are important in the maintenance of pain often form part of a multimodal pain therapy (Kohlert, Wick, and Rosendahl, 2021). AT is frequently included as a part of a multimodal therapeutic approach to pain management (Sadigh, 2001). In Germany, where almost every healthcare facility provides some form of multimodal pain treatment, AT is widely used alongside relaxation techniques.

Kohlert, A., Wick, K., and Rosendahl, J. (2021). Autogenic Training for Reducing Chronic Pain: a Systematic Review and Meta-analysis of Randomized Controlled Trials. *Int. J. Behav. Med.* doi: 10.1007/s12529-021-10038-6.

Miu, A., Renata, M. H., and Mirclea, M. (2009). Reduced Heart Rate Variability and Vagal Tone in Anxiety: Trait Versus State, and the Effects of Autogenic Training, *Autonomic Neuroscience: Basic and Clinical.* 145(1–2), pp. 99–103. doi: 10.1016/j.autneu.2008.11.010.

Sadigh, M. R. (2001). *Autogenic Training: A Mind-Body Approach to the Treatment of Fibromyalgia and Chronic Pain Syndrome.* Boca Raton: CRC Press.

Case study 2—high blood pressure
John, age 65, was referred by his GP. John desperately needed to reduce his blood pressure but was having an adverse reaction to blood pressure medication.

At his GP's request, John met with an AT practitioner who began by completing the medical questionnaire with John as well as taking his blood pressure. John agreed to learn the six AT standard exercises. Over a six-week period with the AT practitioner taking John's blood pressure at the beginning and end of each session, there appeared to be a significant reduction in his systolic pressure as well as a reduction in his diastolic pressure. The phrase (organ-specific formula) John found most helpful was 'my heartbeat is calm and regular'.

John's AT training was straightforward, and the AT practitioner reported back to his GP after three weeks AT training and again at the end of six weeks of training. After completing the eight-week course, John then continued AT practice as part of his daily routine, maintaining his blood pressure at a lower, healthier range.

Kanji, N., White, A., and Ernst, E. (1999). Anti-Hypertensive Effects of Autogenic Training: A Systemic Review, *Perfusion*, 12, pp. 279–282.

Watanabe, Y., Cornélissen, G., Watanabe, M., Watanabe, F., Otsuka, K., Ohkawa, S., Kikuchi, T., and Halberg, F. (2003). Effects of Autogenic Training and Antihypertensive Agents on Circadian and Circaseptan Variation of Blood Pressure, *Clinical and Experimental Hypertension*, 25(7), pp. 405–412. doi: 10.1081/CEH-120024984.

Case study 3—idiopathic Reynaud's disease with vasospastic attacks
Sylvia, age 49, was referred for AT training by a consultant rheumatologist who was hopeful that learning Autogenics could help Sylvia gain more control of her skin temperature. If she could gain some sense of being in charge of herself, the consultant hoped that with an increased sense of her own agency the frequency and intensity of

the vasospastic attacks Sylvia suffered could reduce. A vasospastic attack is an episodic spasm which causes the small blood vessels in the fingers and toes to constrict in response to temperature extremes or emotional intensity resulting in extreme pain.

Sylvia learnt the six AT standard exercises over a six-week period, and then, with the help of an AT practitioner, began to focus on her hands which were particularly vulnerable to attacks of severe cold. The phrase (organ-specific formula) Sylvia found most helpful was 'my hands and feet are warm'. Sylvia responded really well over a period of three months and noticed a significant change in her ability to manage the vasospastic attacks. This in turn improved her feeling of emotional wellbeing as she was able to feel more in charge of herself. She also reported feeling generally calmer. Learning and practising Autogenics did not cure Sylvia's idiopathic Reynaud's disease but her AT practice made her life a bit more comfortable physically as well as mentally.

Stetter, F. and Kupper, S. (2002). Autogenic Training: A Meta-Analysis of Clinical Outcome Studies, *Appl. Psychophysiol. Biofeedback*, 27, pp. 45–98. doi: 10.1023/A:1014576505223.

Surwit, R., Pilon, R., and Fenton, C. (1978). Behavioral Treatment of Raynaud's Disease. *Journal of Behavioral Medicine*, 1, pp. 323–335. doi: 10.1007/BF00846683.

Case study 4—anxiety

Briony, age 56, was referred by her GP for autogenic training because she did not want pharmaceutical treatment for her generalised anxiety state. Briony had a stressful career as a banker and was an older mother of two children aged 16 and 13 years. She had become increasingly anxious about her daily life, worrying that she might lose her job and being fearful that her children would get very ill. Briony described herself as constantly feeling anxious, suffering from nausea, feeling out of control, and struggling to get to sleep.

The AT practitioner completed a medical questionnaire with Briony, who then agreed to attend weekly sessions to learn the six AT standard exercises. The AT practitioner helped her note the key anxiety issues and graded them on a scale of 1–10. In Week 1, Briony's subjective score was 8/9 (high anxiety). Over the weeks of learning AT, this scale was monitored by the AT practitioner to see how Briony progressed.

Briony struggled with the first few AT sessions due to not being able to concentrate on the AT formula. When Briony agreed with her AT practitioner that she needed to set aside specific 'Briony time' for her AT practice and also to find quiet places for her practice, Briony's experience of learning AT improved. Briony found adding a phrase (organ-specific formula), 'I sleep quietly and well', helped her attain and maintain good sleep.

After the third week, Briony reported noticing a change in her sleep pattern, describing how she was able to drift off to sleep by repeating the autogenic formulae when in bed.

After week five, Briony noticed she was not 'fretting' as much and hadn't had a deep worry about the children becoming seriously ill for at least five days. Over the course of the eight weeks of AT training, there was a significant reduction in Briony's general anxiety and her subjective scoring of anxiety levels dropped from 8/9 to mostly 3/4.

Briony continued with the AT practice and built AT into her life. In a review six months later, she was still using AT, felt she was able to function better at home and work, and reported feeling more relaxed and happy.

Medical practitioners often refer patients diagnosed with anxiety disorders to AT practitioners as those are the patients who often develop psychosomatic co-morbidity such as high blood pressure or pain in joints due to rheumatoid or osteo-arthritis to name a few (Ernst and Kanji, 2000).

Ernst, E. and Kanji, N. (2000). Autogenic Training for Stress and Anxiety: A Systematic Review, *Complementary Therapies in Medicine*, 8(2), pp. 106–110. doi: 10.1054/ctim.2000.0354.

Kanji, N., White, A. R., and Ernst, E. (2004). Autogenic Training Reduces Anxiety after Coronary Angioplasty: A Randomized

Clinical Trial, *American Heart Journal*, 147(3), pp. 508. doi: 10.1016/j.ahj.2003.10.011.

Time and again, AT practitioners report the reduction or total disappearance of a variety of clinical symptoms in clients suffering from a wide range of medical problems. Autogenic training is effective in bringing about, in a substantially shorter time than many other therapeutic interventions, a greater balance in our body mind system. Over time and with regular daily AT practice, we can develop greater inner self-awareness and become more able to act outwards in the world with greater intention and purpose.

Frequently, the changes in our body mind system that occur as a result of practising AT can happen outside of our conscious awareness and clients do not seem to require much discussion when changes occur. This we believe is because restoring our body mind system to a state of balance is aligned with the way we are designed to thrive and flourish when our parasympathetic nervous system is activated and doing its job of enabling rest, relaxation, repair, and restoration. Too often, our parasympathetic nervous system is highjacked and unable to function as intended because without our even knowing it our sympathetic nervous system is being overactive too much of the time.

Examples of some other medical conditions routinely encountered by medical practitioners, whose patients report finding symptomatic relief from practising AT, are: athletes suffering from performance anxiety, addictions, asthma, cancer—management of symptoms resulting from treatment, chronic health conditions, depression, diabetes, fatigue, heart disease, insomnia, migraine headaches, tension headaches, unexplained and undiagnosed physical pain. AT has been found to significantly relieve symptoms of many different medical conditions. So whilst AT is not a cure for any condition and is not intended to replace standard medical treatments, AT can help people better manage symptoms, thus contributing to an improved quality of life.

In a meta-analysis study of clinical outcomes, Stetter and Kupper (2002) noted the following physical, emotional, and psychological benefits of Autogenics:

- Headache relief: a 2018 review found autogenic training to be helpful in decreasing headache pain.
- Researchers have found that autogenic training is helpful in managing symptoms and psychological distress in people living with chronic health problems.
- Anxiety relief: researchers discovered autogenic training had a direct and positive impact on anxiety.
- Anxiety and stress relief following medical procedures: people who learnt and used autogenic training in addition to their regular medical care seem to experience less anxiety following a heart procedure than those who had not learnt and used Autogenics after surgery. The group using autogenic training also reported an increase in their overall quality of life.
- Improvement in depression and anxiety symptoms: Some studies have shown that participants living with depression and/or anxiety who use AT benefit by having a reduction in their symptoms.

Carruthers, M. (1979). Autogenic Training. *J. Psychosom. Res.*, 23(6), pp. 437–440. doi: 10.1016/0022-3999(79)90059-X.

Kanji, N. (2000). Management of Pain Through Autogenic Training. *Complement. Ther. Nurs. Midwifery*, 6(3), pp. 143–148. doi: 10.1054/ctnm.2000.0473.

Luthe, W. (1963). Autogenic Training: Method, Research and Application in Medicine. *Am. J. Psychother.*, 17, pp. 174–195. doi: 10.1176/appi.psychotherapy.1963.17.2.174.

Pikoff, H. (1984). A critical review of autogenic training in America. *Clin. Psychol. Rev.*, 4(6), pp. 619–639. doi: 10.1016/0272-7358(84)90009-6.

Schultz, J. H. (1932). *Das autogene Training (konzentrative Selbstentspannung). Versuch einer klinisch-praktischen Darstellung.* Leipzig: G. Thieme.

Stetter, F. and Kupper, S. (2002). Autogenic training: a meta-analysis of clinical outcome studies. *Appl Psychophysiol. Biofeedback*, 27(1), pp. 45–98. doi: 10.1023/A:1014576505223.

Autogenic training medical questionnaire

The answers to the following questions are important in planning your course of autogenic training. The answers you give will be treated in the strictest confidence.

Take your time filling details. Go over the form several times. If you are uncertain as to how to answer a question, put a question mark.

Name: .... DOB: ....

Single/Married/Divorced/Separated

Address:..

....

....

Occupation: ....

Schooling: Primary School .... years

Secondary School: .... years

Higher Education .... years

Religious education to the age of 12 ....

Section 1: Your health history

Have you ever had any of these illnesses, either now or in the past?

Tick if the answer is yes.

Allergies or asthma:	....	Heart trouble:	....
Diabetes:	....	Epilepsy/Fits:	....
Stomach Ulcers:	....	Chronic Indigestion:	....

High blood pressure: ....   Glaucoma: ....

Kidney trouble: ....   Bladder trouble: ....

Rheumatism: ....   Arthritis: ....

Drug addiction: ....   Drug dependence: ....

Nervous breakdown: ....   Anxiety: ....

Sleep problems: ....

Give details: ....

....

....

....

Section 2: Medicines

Give details of any medicines you are taking now and any medicines you are allergic to:

....

....

To help jog your memory:

Antacids	Sedatives	Sleeping Pills
Tranquilisers	Blood Pressure	Antidepressants
Contraceptives	Laxatives	

Have you ever used non-prescribed drugs?
LSD, marijuana, cocaine, heroin, amphetamines, glue or any other drugs

Yes .... No ....

Give details: ....

Section 3: Family history

Relative	Present state of health	Date of Death	Cause of Death
Mother	....	....	....
Father	....	....	....
Brothers/Sisters	....	....	....
	....	....	....
Children	....	....	....
	....	....	....
Grandparents	....	....	....

Section 4: Operations and medical procedures

Make a note here of any operations or medical procedures you have undergone, followed by your age (approximately) at the time:

To jog your memory:
Tonsils, appendix, gall bladder, hysterectomy, vasectomy, sterilisation, spinal tap, dental surgery, mastectomy

Give details: ....

....

....

Were any of these particularly unpleasant experiences?

....

....

Have you had any unpleasant experiences involving anaesthetics?

....

....

Have you suffered from bleeding or haemorrhage where you needed a transfusion or drip?

....

....

Have you ever been in hospital for a serious illness or operation (apart from pregnancy)?

....

....

Have you had any other illness or treatment not mentioned above?

....

....

Section 5: Alterations of consciousness

Please tick if the answer is yes.

Have you ever experienced a change in consciousness?

a) From being hypnotised   ....

b) From taking drugs   ....

c) From alcohol   ....

d) From an overdose   ....

e) From inhaling smoke, gas
or exhaust fumes   ....
f) From nearly drowning   ....
g) Other   ....

Section 6: Emotional disturbances

Please tick if the answer is yes.

Have you:

a) Ever been seriously emotionally
disturbed   ....
b) Felt that your body was unreal   ....
c) Felt intensely agitated or
depressed   ....
d) Suffered from phobias   ....
e) Suffered from panics   ....

Have you ever consulted a psychiatrist or
psychotherapist: YES/NO
Have you ever had outpatient or inpatient
treatment in a psychiatric unit?   YES/NO

Section 7: Your birth

Were there any complications in the pregnancy?   YES/NO
Was the birth difficult?   YES/NO
Were you premature?   YES/NO
Were you born late?   YES/NO
Were you breast fed?   YES/NO

Section 8: Accidents and injuries

Please write details of any serious accidents or injuries you have had, particularly where there were alterations of consciousness from loss of blood, fainting or head

To jog your memory:

Sports injuries, traffic accidents, fires, falls, tools and machinery, head injuries, being chased, amusement parks

Your age   **Nature of accident or injury**

....

....

....

....

Section 9: Your lifestyle

Please answer Yes or No to all these questions:

a)	Do you drive to work?	YES/NO
b)	Are you overweight?	YES/NO
c)	Do you smoke?	YES/NO
d)	Do you regularly drink alcohol?	YES/NO
e)	Do you regularly work long hours?	YES/NO
f)	Does your job involve working to deadlines?	YES/NO
g)	Do you take regular exercise?	YES/NO

What sort of exercise do you take?

....

....

....

....

Section 10: Your personality

Please tick any question where your answer is Yes

Are you eager to compete?   ....

Are you a driving, forceful person?   ....

Are you anxious for recognition at work

or in any other setting?   ....

Are you conscious of time and deadlines?   ....

Do you have to win when you play games?   ....

Are you made angry by things or people?   ....

Do you have problems with anger?   ....

Are you an impatient person?   ....

Do you need to get things done quickly?   ....

Do you undertake a lot of different activities?   ....

Do you find it difficult to say 'No' when you

need to?   ....

Do you stop yourself crying when you need

to cry?   ....

Did your religious education ever trouble you?

Frequently: .... Occasionally: .... Never: ....

Section 11: Your overall view of your life

Answer these five questions are you feel now, today.

Answer them on a scale of 0—20 (0 = not at all, 20 = entirely)

a) How far do you feel you have achieved

your aims in life?   ....

b) How far do you feel hopeful

for the future?   ....

c) How far do you feel your life

has meaning?   ....

d) How far has life given you scope

for self-expression?   ....

e) When you look back, how far do you feel

life has been worth the struggle? ....

If there is anything else you would like to add about your health or lifestyle, please write below:

....

....

....

....

Section 12: Female problems

Men should omit this section and go directly to the end of the questionnaire.

Is your menstrual cycle regular? ....

How long do your periods last? ....

Are your periods regular or irregular? ....

Do you suffer from or have you suffered from:

a) Painful periods?   YES/NO

b) Heavy periods?   YES/NO

c) Lack of periods?   YES/NO

d) Premenstrual tension?   YES/NO

e) Has your fertility ever caused you anxiety?   YES/NO

Please give details of any pregnancies you have had:

Your age	Length of pregnancy (Months)	Live/ stillbirth	Type of delivery (forceps, caesarean, normal)

....

....

....

Were there problems during any of your pregnancies or births? Give details:

....

....

....

....

....

Did you have difficulties with post-natal depression or emotional difficulties?

....

....

Were there any difficulties with the baby in the first few months?

....

....

Declaration:
I have answered this questionnaire to the best of my knowledge and recollection.

.... **Name**

CONCLUSION

Our aim in writing this book has been to make autogenic training (AT) available to a wider public in a format that enables people to teach themselves the six AT standard exercises created by Johannes Schulz in the 1920s. Schulz's vision, which was for autogenic training (AT) to be a self-help skillset that people could learn and use without the need for the involvement of a healthcare professional, has been a driver for us.

We have said that with the stresses of life in the 21st century, heightened during the COVID-19 pandemic followed by the war in Ukraine, it has become imperative that people concerned about maintaining their health and resilience and disease prevention who have neither time nor money to work with a qualified AT practitioner have direct access to a skillset like AT. The six AT standard exercises enable us at any time to restore our body mind system to a state of balance (homeostasis) so that our stress response (SNS) is turned off and rest and repair (PSNS) is turned on.

We have written about the history and development of AT around the world on all five continents showing how AT has been adapted by both the local self-care cultures and medical practices, even becoming mainstream in some countries.

In addition to the six AT standard exercises, we have given examples of how AT can complement conventional medicine and is used successfully for treating a variety of medical conditions, thus often reducing the need for both pharmaceutical interventions and medical practitioners' time. So if you ever want to explore whether AT can bring relief to a specific medical condition, you will need to work with a qualified AT practitioner. Working together with a qualified AT practitioner, you will be able to design organ-specific formulae or personal motivational formulae unique to your health needs. When you know from your expanded AT practice that the formulae created in collaboration with your AT-qualified practitioner are helping relieve or dissolve your symptoms, you will be able to continue your AT expanded practise without needing further help from an outside person apart from occasional monitoring of how you are progressing.

By now, we hope you are feeling the benefits of having set aside the time to learn the six AT standard exercises and hope you look forward to and enjoy knowing that your daily AT practice enhances your resilience, and strengthens and supports your immune system. Once part of your daily routine, you can be confident that your daily practise is providing you with the means to restore your body mind system to a state of balance (homeostasis). You will have learnt how to access the relaxation response and how to allow your body mind system to self-regulate.

We have been clear that whilst some people do report finding AT becomes their preferred and effective alternative to taking medication for stress-related symptoms, AT is not a replacement for conventional medicine. Also, we have identified certain health conditions for which AT may be contraindicated and should then only be learnt with a qualified AT practitioner who can carefully monitor a person's responses when learning the six AT standard exercises.

Finally, we cannot emphasise enough the benefits of making AT a daily habit. AT allows us to offload stress, anxiety, and physical tensions. Restoring calm, focus, and general wellbeing. It is clear to us and hopefully now to you that AT has an important part to play in preventative medicine. We would welcome feedback about this book and any questions you have about AT, so please do feel free to contact us (gaylin@5tconsulting.net or rosdraper@crisalida.co.uk).

Wishing you many happy years of using the six AT standard exercises!

HOW TO LEARN MORE ABOUT AT AND ACCESS QUALIFIED AT PRACTITIONERS

In this section, we provide information about how and where to find qualified AT practitioners as well as listing material available both online and from bookstores

Visit the websites of the British Autogenic Society (www.autogenic-therapy.org.uk) and the International Society of Autogenic Training and Psychotherapy (www.isatapsy.com), where you will find many free resources as well as links for finding AT practitioners worldwide.

On the website of Dr Ian Ross (www.atdynamics.co.uk), an experienced Autogenic Trainer, you will also find a wealth of resources.

Books

The Relaxation Response: Herbert Benson (1975 and reissued 2000).
Autogenic Training—The Effective Holistic Way To Better Health: Kai Kermani (1997), Souvenir Press Limited.
Autogenic Therapy—Self-Help for Mind and Body: Jane Bird and Christine Pinch (2002), New Leaf.
Autogenics 3.0—The New Way to Mindfulness and Meditation: Luis de Rivera (2nd edition 2018 revised), ICAT.

Introductory Workshop—Methods of Autogenic Training: Wolfgang Luthe and Luis de Rivera (2015), ICAT.

Autogenic training: A Mind-Body Approach to the Treatment of Chronic Pain Syndrome and Stress-Related Disorders: Micah R. Sadigh (3rd edition 2019), McFarland Health Topics.

REFERENCES

Benson, H. and Klipper, M.Z. (2000). *The relaxation response*. New York: Wings Books.

Carruthers, M. (1979). Autogenic training. *Journal of Psychosomatic Research*, 23(6), pp. 437–440. doi:10.1016/0022-3999(79)90059-x.

De Rivera, L. (2005). *Crisis Emocionales*. Madrid: Espasa.

De Rivera, L. (Ed.), (2015). *Wolfgang Luthe: Introductory Workshop to the Methods of Autogenic Therapy*. Scotts Valley, California: CreateSpace Independent Publishing. Vol 1.

De Rivera, L. (2017). *Autogenics 3.0*. Scotts Valley, California: Createspace Independent Publishing Platform.

Ernst, E. and Kanji, N. (2000). Autogenic training for stress and anxiety: A systematic review. *Complementary Therapies in Medicine*, 8(2), pp. 106–110. doi:10.1054/ctim.2000.0354.

Kanji, A., White, A.R. and Ernst, E. (1999). Anti-hypertensive effects of autogenic training: A systematic review. *Perfusion*, 12(7), pp. 279–282.

Kanji, N., White, A.R. and Ernst, E. (2004). Autogenic training reduces anxiety after coronary angioplasty: A randomized clinical trial. *American Heart Journal*, 147(3), p. 508. doi:10.1016/j.ahj.2003.10.011.

Kanji, N. (2000). Management of pain through autogenic training. *Complementary Therapies in Nursing and Midwifery*, 6(3), pp. 143–148. doi:10.1054/ctnm.2000.0473.

Kermani, K. (2009). *Autogenic training: The effective holistic way to better health*. London: Souvenir Press Limited

Luthe, W. (1963). Autogenic Training: Method, Research and Application in Medicine. *American Journal of Psychotherapy*, 17(2), pp. 174–195. doi:10.1176/appi.psychotherapy.1963.17.2.174.

Luthe, W. and Schultz. J.H. (1969). *Autogenic Therapy*. Edited by W. Luthe. New York: Grune & Stratton. Vol. 1, Porges, S.W. (2007). The polyvagal perspective. *Biological Psychology*, 74(2), pp. 116–143. doi:10.1016/j.biopsycho.2006.06.009.

Porges, S.W. (2009). The Polyvagal Theory: New Insights into Adaptive Reactions of the Autonomic Nervous System. *Cleveland Clinic Journal of Medicine*, [online] 76(Suppl_2), pp. 86–90. doi:10.3949/ccjm.76.s2.17.

Porges, S.W. (2011). *The polyvagal theory: Neurophysiological foundations of emotions, attachment, communication, and self-regulation*. New York: Norton.

Porges, S.W. (2017). *The pocket guide to polyvagal theory: The transformative power of feeling safe*. New York, N.Y.: W.W. Norton & Company.

Porges, S.W. and Dana, D. (2018). *Clinical Applications of the Polyvagal Theory: The emergence of polyvagal-informed therapies*. New York: W. W. Norton & Company, Inc.

Sadigh, M.R. (2020). *Autogenic Training: A Mind-Body Approach to the Treatment of Chronic Pain Syndrome and Stress-Related Disorders*. North Carolina: McFarland & Company.

Sadigh, M.R. (2020). 'Lecture given to BAS Foundation Course' [Lecture] 12 March.

Stetter, F. and Kupper, S. (2002). Autogenic training: A meta-analysis of clinical outcome studies. *Applied Psychophysiology and Biofeedback*, 27(1), pp. 45–98. doi:10.1023/a:1014576505223.

Surwit, R.S., Pilon, R.N. and Fenton, C.H. (1978). Behavioral treatment of Raynaud's disease. *Journal of Behavioral Medicine*, 1(3), pp. 323–335. doi:10.1007/bf00846683.

Watanabe, Y. *et al.* (2003). Effects of Autogenic Training and Anti-hypertensive Agents on Circadian and Circaseptan Variation of Blood Pressure. *Clinical and Experimental Hypertension*, 25(7), pp. 405–412. doi:10.1081/ceh-120024984.

FURTHER READING

ATdynamics. (2020). Autogenic Switches and Well-being. Available at: https://atdynamics.co.uk/wp-content/uploads/2020/07/B-24-Autogenic-Switches-and-Well-Being-2020.pdf.

Bird, J. and Pinch, C. (2002). *Autogenic Therapy*. Dublin: New Leaf.

Bowlby, J. (1952). *Maternal Care and Mental Health: A Report Prepared on Behalf of the World Health Organization as a Contribution to the United Nations Programme for the Welfare of Homeless Children*. World Health Organization.

Bowlby, J. (1969–1980). *Attachment and loss*. (3 Volumes), London: Pimlico.

Bowlby, J. (1988). *A secure base: Clinical application of attachment theory*. London: Tavistock-Routledge.

Buckner, R.L., Andrews-Hanna, J.R. and Schacter, D.L. (2008). The Brain's Default Network. *Annals of the New York Academy of Sciences*, 1124(1), pp. 1–38. doi:10.1196/annals.1440.011.

Cannon, W.B. (1915). *Bodily changes in pain, hunger, fear and rage: An account of recent researches into the function of emotional excitement*. New York: D Appleton & Company. doi:10.1037/10013-000.

Cannon, W.B. (1932). *The wisdom of the body*. New York: W.W. Norton & Co.

Cannon, W.B. (1936). The role of emotion in disease. *Annals of Internal medicine*, 9(11), pp. 1453–1465.

Capra, F. and Luigi, P L. (2018). *The systems view of life: A unifying vision*. New York: Cambridge University Press.

Chugani, H.T., *et al*. (2001). Local Brain Functional Activity Following Early Deprivation: A Study of Postinstitutionalized Romanian Orphans. *NeuroImage*, 14(6), pp. 1290–1301. doi:10.1006/nimg.2001.0917.

Clarivate Analytics. (2016). *Citation Classics 1986*. Available at: http://garfield.library.upenn.edu/classics1986/A1986F062900001.pdf

Craig, A.D. (2005). Forebrain emotional asymmetry: A neuroanatomical basis? *Trends in cognitive sciences*, 9(12), pp. 566–571.

Craig, A.D. (2013). Cooling, pain, and other feelings from the body in relation to the autonomic nervous system. *Autonomic Nervous System*, pp. 103–109. doi:10.1016/b978-0-444-53491-0.00009-2.

Craig, A.D. (2014). *How Do You Feel? An Interoceptive Moment with your Neurobiological Self*. New Jersey: Princeton University Press.

Creswell, J.D., *et al*. (2007). Neural Correlates of Dispositional Mindfulness During Affect Labeling. *Psychosomatic Medicine*, 69(6), pp. 560–565. doi:10.1097/psy.0b013e3180f6171f.

Creswell, J.D. and Lindsay, E.K. (2014). How Does Mindfulness Training Affect Health? A Mindfulness Stress Buffering Account. *Current Directions in Psychological Science*, 23(6), pp. 401–407. doi:10.1177/0963721414547415.

Csikszentmihalyi, M. (2002). *Flow: The Psychology of Happiness*. London: Ebury Publishing.

Damasio, A.R. (1994). *Descartes' error: Emotion, reason, and the human brain*. New York: Putnam.

Damasio, A.R. (2000). The *Feeling of what happens: Body and emotion in the making of consciousness*. Boston: Mariner Books.

Damasio, A.R. (2004). *Looking for Spinoza: Joy, sorrow, and the feeling brain*. London: Vintage.

Davidson, R.J., *et al*. (2003). Alterations in Brain and Immune Function Produced by Mindfulness Meditation. *Psychosomatic Medicine*, 65(4), pp. 564–570. doi:10.1097/01.psy.0000077505.67574.e3.

Davidson, R.J. (2003). 'The Neuroscience of Emotion', in D. Goleman (Ed.), *A Dialogue with the Dalai Lama: Destructive Emotions and how we can overcome them*. London: Bloomsbury pp. 179–204.

Davidson, R.J. (2005). Emotion regulation, happiness, and the neuroplasticity of the brain. *Advances in Mind-Body Medicine*, 21(3–4), 25–28.

Davidson, R.J. and Begley, S. (2013). *The emotional life of your brain: How its unique patterns affect the way you think, feel, and live—and how you can change them.* New York: Plume.

Delgado, M.R., *et al.* (2008). Neural Circuitry Underlying the Regulation of Conditioned Fear and Its Relation to Extinction. *Neuron*, 59(5), pp. 829–838. doi:10.1016/j.neuron.2008.06.029.

Dingham, M. (2014). *Know your brain: Prefrontal cortex.* Available at: https://neuroscientificallychallenged.com/posts/know-your-brain-prefrontal-cortex (Accessed: 13 April 2020).

Dobbin, A. and Ross, S. (2012). Resilience and recovery: Dumping dualism. *Contemporary Hypnosis & Integrative Therapy*, 29(2), pp. 136–155.

Ekman, P., *et al.* (2005). Buddhist and Psychological Perspectives on Emotions and Well-Being. *Current Directions in Psychological Science*, 14(2), pp. 59–63. doi:10.1111/j.0963-7214.2005.00335.x.

Frankl, V.E. (1997). *Man's search for meaning.* London: Pocket Books.

Frankl, V.E. (2012). *The Doctor and the Soul.* London: Souvenir Press.

Fredrickson, B.L. (2001). The role of positive emotions in positive psychology: The broaden-and-build theory of positive emotions. *American Psychologist*, 56(3), pp. 218–226. doi:10.1037/0003-066x.56.3.218.

Fredrickson, B.L., *et al.* (2000). The Undoing Effect of Positive Emotions. *Motivation and Emotion*, 24(4), pp. 237–258. doi:10.1023/a:1010796329158.

Fredrickson, B. (2003). The Value of Positive Emotions. *American Scientist*, 91(4), pp. 330–335. doi:10.1511/2003.4.330.

Fredrickson, B. (2009). *Positivity.* New York: Harmony Books.

Gaete, H.P. (2016). Hypothalamus-pituitary-adrenal (HPA) axis, chronic stress, hair cortisol, metabolic syndrome and mindfulness. *Integrative Molecular Medicine*, 3(5). doi:10.15761/imm.1000244.

Garrison, K.A., *et al.* (2015). Meditation leads to reduced default mode network activity beyond an active task. *Cognitive, Affective, & Behavioral Neuroscience*, [online] 15(3), pp. 712–720. doi:10.3758/s13415-015-0358-3.

Gilbert, P. (2009). *The compassionate mind: A new approach to life's challenges.* London: Robinson.

Gilbert, P. and Choden. (2013). *Mindful compassion: Using the power of mindfulness and compassion to transform our lives.* London: Robinson.

Goleman, D. (2003). *Destructive Emotions: A dialogue with The Dalai Lama narrated.* New York: Bantam.

Gordon, J.S. (1996). *Manifesto For A New Medicine.* Cambridge, USA: Da Capo Lifelong Books.

Graham, L. (2019). *Resilience: Powerful practices for bouncing back from disappointment, difficulty, and even disaster.* California: New World Library.

Griffin, J., Tyrrell, I. and Farouk, O. (2015). *Human givens: The new approach to emotional health and clear thinking.* Chalvington: Human Givens.

Hanh, T.N. (1990). *Our Appointment with Life: Discourse on Living Happily in the Present Moment.* Translated from the Vietnamese by A. Laity. California: Parallax Press.

Hanh, T.N. (1990). *Present moment, wonderful moment: Mindfulness verses for daily living.* California: Parallax Press.

Hanh, T.N. (2015). *The heart of the Buddha's teaching: Transforming suffering into peace, joy & liberation.* New York: Harmony Books.

Hanh, T.N. and Mcleod, M. (2012). *The pocket Thich Nhat Hanh.* Boston: Shambhala.

Hanh, T.N. (2015). *Silence: The Power of Quiet in a World Full of Noise.* New York: Harper Collins.

Hanh, T.N. (2017). *The Other Shore: A New Translation of the Heart Sutra with Commentaries.* California: Palm Leaves Press.

Harlow, H.F., Dodsworth, R.O. and Harlow, M.K. (1965). Total Social Isolation in Monkeys. *Proceedings of the National Academy of Sciences,* [online] 54(1), pp. 90–97. doi:10.1073/pnas.54.1.90.

Henry, J.P. (1987). Psychological Factors and Coronary Heart Disease. *Holistic Medicine,* 2(3), pp. 119–132. doi:10.3109/13561828709043570.

Hill, S. (1974). *In the Springtime of the Year.* Boston: David R. Godine.

House, J. (1981). *Work, Stress, and Social Support.* New York, Addison-Wesley.

Iaccino, J.F. (2014). *Left Brain-Right Brain Differences*. London: Psychology Press.

Kabat-Zinn, J. (1990). *Full catastrophe living: Using the wisdom of your body and mind to face stress, pain, and illness*. New York: Dell Publishing Co.

Isen, A.M. (2008). 'Some ways in which positive affect influences decision making and problem solving.' In M. Lewis, J.M. Haviland-Jones, and L.F. Barrett (Eds.), *Handbook of emotions*. New York: The Guilford Press pp. 548–573.

Kang, D.-H., *et al.* (2012). The effect of meditation on brain structure: Cortical thickness mapping and diffusion tensor imaging. *Social Cognitive and Affective Neuroscience*, [online] 8(1), pp. 27–33. doi:10.1093/scan/nss056.

Karasek, R.A. (1979). Job Demands, Job Decision Latitude, and Mental Strain: Implications for Job Redesign. *Administrative Science Quarterly*, 24(2), pp. 285–308. doi:10.2307/2392498.

Karasek, R.A., *et al.* (1988). Job characteristics in relation to the prevalence of myocardial infarction in the US Health Examination Survey (HES) and the Health and Nutrition Examination Survey (HANES). *American Journal of Public Health*, 78(8), pp. 910–918. doi:10.2105/ajph.78.8.910.

Killingsworth, M.A. and Gilbert, D.T. (2010). A Wandering Mind Is an Unhappy Mind. *Science*, [online] 330(6006), pp. 932–932. doi:10.1126/science.1192439.

Kohlert, A., Wick, K. and Rosendahl, J. (2021). Autogenic Training for Reducing Chronic Pain: A Systematic Review and Meta-analysis of Randomized Controlled Trials. *International Journal of Behavioral Medicine*. doi:10.1007/s12529-021-10038-6.

Kringelbach, M.L. (2004). 'Emotion', in R.L. Gregory (Ed.), *The Oxford Companion to the Mind*. Oxford: Oxford University Press.

Landon, H.C R. (1992). *Beethoven: His Life, Work and World*. London: Thames and Hudson.

Levine, P. (2018). 'Polyvagal Theory and Trauma', in S. Porges and D. Dana (Ed.), *Clinical Applications of the Polyvagal Theory*. New York: W.W. Norton & Company, pp. 3–26.

Ledoux, J. (1999). *The Emotional Brain The Mysterious Underpinnings of Emotional Life*. London: Weidenfeld & Nicolson.

Lieberman, M.D., *et al.* (2007). Putting feelings into words: Affect labeling disrupts amygdala activity in response to affective stimuli. *Psychological Science*, [online] 18(5), pp. 421–428. doi:10.1111/j.1467-9280.2007.01916.x.

Luders, E., *et al.* (2009). The underlying anatomical correlates of long-term meditation: Larger hippocampal and frontal volumes of gray matter. *Neurolmage*, 45(3), pp. 672–678. doi:10.1016/j.neuroimage.2008.12.061.

Lyubomirsky, S., Sheldon, K.M. and Schkade, D. (2005). Pursuing happiness: The architecture of sustainable change. *Review of General Psychology*, [online] 9(2), pp. 111–131. doi:10.1037/1089-2680.9.2.111.

Maslow, A.H. (1954). *Motivation and personality.* 3rd ed. New York: Addison Wesley Longman.

Maslow, A.H. (1982). *Toward a psychology of being.* New York: Van Nostrand Reinhold.

Mate.Gabor. (2011). When the Body says No, Penguin.

Medicinska Fakulteten vid LiU () *How do you feel? Lecture by Bud Craig.* 14 December. Available at: https://vimeo.com/8170544.

McEwen, B.S. (1998). Protective and Damaging Effects of Stress Mediators. *New England Journal of Medicine*, 338(3), pp. 171–179. doi:10.1056/nejm199801153380307.

McEwen, B. and Lasley, E.N. (2003). Allostatic load: When protection gives way to damage. *Adv Mind Body Med*, 19(1), pp. 28–33.

McEwen, B.S. (2004). 'Protective and Damaging Effects of the Mediators of Stress and Adaptation: Allostasis and Allostatic Load', in J. Schulkin (Ed.), *Allostasis, Homeostasis, and the costs of adaptation.* Cambridge: Cambridge University Press, pp. 65–91.

Mcgilchrist, I. (2019). *MASTER AND HIS EMISSARY: The divided brain and the making of the western world.* New Haven: Yale University Press.

Miu, A.C., Heilman, R.M. and Miclea, M. (2009). Reduced heart rate variability and vagal tone in anxiety: Trait versus state, and the effects of autogenic training. *Autonomic Neuroscience*, 145(1–2), pp. 99–103. doi:10.1016/j.autneu.2008.11.010.

Needham, J. (1956). *Science and Civilisation in China: History of Scientific Thought: History of Scientific Thought.* Vol 2. Cambridge: Cambridge University Press.

Ngomane, M. (2019). *Everyday Ubuntu: Living better together, the African way*. London: Transworld Digital.

Nscience. (n.d.). *Vagus Nerve Regulation and Trauma Recovery: Video Course*. [online] Available at: https://www.nscience.uk/product/vagus-nerve-regulation-and-trauma-recovery/ [Accessed November 2022].

Pace-Schott, E.F. and Picchioni, D. (2017). Neurobiology of Dreaming. *Principles and Practice of Sleep Medicine*, pp. 529–538.e6. doi:10.1016/b978-0-323-24288-2.00051-9.

Panksepp, J. (2005). *Affective Neuroscience: The Foundations of Human and Animal Emotions*. Oxford, New York: Oxford University Press.

Panksepp, J. (2009). 'Brain Emotional Systems and Qualities of Mental Life', in D. Fosha, D. Siegel and M. Solomon (Ed.), *The Healing Power of Emotion*. New York: W.W. Norton & Company, pp. 1–26.

Panksepp, J. Biven, L. and Siegel, D.J. (2012). *The archaeology of mind: Neuroevolutionary origins of human emotions*. New York: W.W. Norton & Co.

Pert, C.B. (1997). *Molecules of Emotion*. New York: Scribner.

Pollard, I. (2004). 'Meditation and Brain function: A review', *Eubios Journal of Asian and International Bioethics*, 14(1), pp. 28–33.

Popescu, S. (2014). Nonlocality beyond quantum mechanics. *Nature Physics*, [online] 10(4), pp. 264–270. doi:10.1038/nphys2916.

Pikoff, H. (1984). A critical review of autogenic training in America. *Clinical Psychology Review*, 4(6), pp. 619–639. doi:10.1016/0272-7358(84)90009-6.

Raichle, M.E., *et al.* (2001). A default mode of brain function. *Proceedings of the National Academy of Sciences*, 98(2), pp. 676–682. doi:10.1073/pnas.98.2.676.

Ross, I. (2010). *Autogenic dynamics: Stress, affect regulation, and autogenic therapy: A selection of essays for therapists and students*. Scotland: Ian Ross.

Rossi, E.L. (2002). *The psychobiology of gene expression: Neuroscience and neurogenesis in hypnosis and the healing arts*. New York: W.W. Norton & Co.

Ryan, R.M. and Deci, E.L. (2000). Self-Determination Theory and the Facilitation of Intrinsic Motivation, Social Development, and Well-Being. *American Psychologist*, 55(1), pp. 68–78.

Spinoza, B.D. (1677). *Ethics*. Translated from the latin by E. Curley. London: Penguin.

Sapolsky, R.M. (2007). 'Stress, Stress-Related Disease, and Emotional Regulation', in J.J. Gross (Ed.), *Handbook of Emotion Regulation*. New York: Guilford Press, pp. 605–615.

Schlamann, M., *et al.* (2010). Autogenic Training Alters Cerebral Activation Patterns in fMRI. *International Journal of Clinical and Experimental Hypnosis*, 58(4), pp. 444–456. doi:10.1080/0020714 4.2010.499347.

Segal, Z.V., *et al.* (2013). *Mindfulness-based cognitive therapy for depression*. New York; London: Guilford Press.

Seligman, M.E.P. (2006). *Learned Optimism: How To Change Your Mind And Your Life*. New York: Vintage Books, C.

Selye, H. (1984). *The stress of life*. New York: McGraw Hill.

Siegel, D.J. (2007). *The Mindful Brain: Reflection and Attunement in the Cultivation of Well-Being (Norton Series on Interpersonal Neurobiology)*. New York: W.W. Norton & Co.

Siegel, D.J. (2010). *The mindful therapist: A clinician's guide to mindsight and neural integration*. New York: W.W. Norton & Co.

Siegel, D.J. (2011). *Mindsight: Transform your brain with the new science of kindness*. London: Oneworld Publications.

Southwick, S.M. and Charney, D. (2018). *Resilience: The science of mastering life's greatest challenges*. Cambridge: Cambridge University Press.

Stellar, J.E., John-Henderson, N., Anderson, C.L., Gordon, A.M., McNeil, G.D. and Keltner, D. (2015). Positive affect and markers of inflammation: Discrete positive emotions predict lower levels of inflammatory cytokines. *Emotion*, 15(2), pp. 129–133. doi:10.1037/emo0000033.

Sterling, P. and Eyer, J. (1988). 'Allostasis: A new paradigm to explain arousal pathology', in S. Fisher & J. Reason (Eds.), *Handbook of life stress, cognition, and health*. New Jersey: Wiley Blackwell, pp. 629–649.

Sterling, P. (2004). 'Principles of Allostasis: Optimal design, predictive regulation, pathophysiology and rational therapeutics', in J. Schulkin (Ed.), *Allostasis, Homeostasis, and the costs of adaptation*. Cambridge: Cambridge University Press, pp. 56–85.

Taft, M. (2017). *Deconstructing Yourself: The Craving Mind, with Judson Brewer* [Podcast]. 24 October. Available at: https://deconstructingyourself.com/dy-009-craving-mind-guest-judson-brewer.html.

TEDx Talks. (2013). *You're Already Awesome. Just Get Out of Your Own Way!: Judson Brewer MD, Ph.D at TEDx RockCreekPark*. 11 May. Available at: https://www.youtube.com/watch?v=jE1j5Om7g0U&ab_channel=TEDxTalks

UNESCO MGIEP. (2018). *Eighth Distinguished Lecture by Prof. Richard Davidson (Complete Video)*. 26 December. https://www.youtube.com/watch?v=lggEMJdk07U&ab_channel=UNESCOMGIE

Van der Kolk. (2020). The body keeps the score, Penguin.

Watts, A. (1995). *The Tao of Philosophy*. Vermont: Tuttle Publishing.

Wei, G. and Luo, J. (2010). Sport expert's motor imagery: Functional imaging of professional motor skills and simple motor skills. *Brain Research*, 1341, pp. 52–62. doi:10.1016/j.brainres.2009.08.014.

Wood, A.M., Froh, J.J. and Geraghty, A.W.A. (2010). Gratitude and well-being: A review and theoretical integration. *Clinical Psychology Review*, 30(7), pp. 890–905. doi:10.1016/j.cpr.2010.03.005.

INDEX

9 781801 520751